D0538421

More Advance Praise for
Cooking with Shelburne Farms

"I've always thought the name Shelburne Farms sells the place short, and now I have proof. *Cooking with Shelburne Farms* shows Shelburne for what it really is: a community, a classroom, an ecological experiment, a showcase for local artisanship . . . a delicious recipe for our time."

—Chef Dan Barber, Blue Hill and Blue Hill at Stone Barns

"This is a terrific book brimming with great stories, pertinent information about ingredients, local history, and well-crafted recipes. We need to support local and seasonal food ways—Melissa and Rick have done so with flavor and style."

—Chef Todd English, Olives

"For more than thirty-five years, Shelburne Farms has pioneered the re-creation of local food webs that bring farmers, children, education, land restoration, and gustatory delights together in order to change our environment for the better. In a book and in practice, Shelburne Farms shows how sustainability can be an act of joy and love."

—Paul Hawken, author of *Blessed Unrest: How the Largest Movement in the World Came into Being and Why No One Saw It Coming*

Cooking *with* Shelburne Farms

Melissa Pasanen

Rick Mullin

Cooking
with
Shelburne
Farms

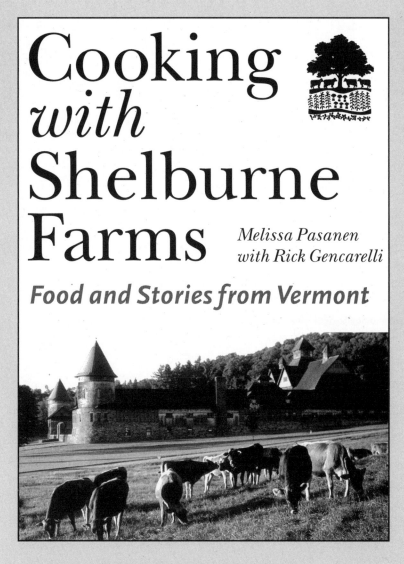

Melissa Pasanen
with Rick Gencarelli

Food and Stories from Vermont

Food photography by Susie Cushner
Portrait photography by Jordan Silverman

Viking Studio

VIKING STUDIO
Published by the Penguin Group
Penguin Group (USA) Inc., 375 Hudson Street,
New York, New York 10014, U.S.A.
Penguin Group (Canada), 90 Eglinton Avenue East, Suite 700,
Toronto, Ontario, Canada M4P 2Y3
(a division of Pearson Penguin Canada Inc.)
Penguin Books Ltd, 80 Strand, London WC2R 0RL, England
Penguin Ireland, 25 St. Stephen's Green, Dublin 2, Ireland
(a division of Penguin Books Ltd)
Penguin Books Australia Ltd, 250 Camberwell Road, Camberwell,
Victoria 3124, Australia
(a division of Pearson Australia Group Pty Ltd)
Penguin Books India Pvt Ltd, 11 Community Centre, Panchsheel Park,
New Delhi – 110 017, India
Penguin Group (NZ), 67 Apollo Drive, Rosedale, North Shore 0632,
New Zealand (a division of Pearson New Zealand Ltd)
Penguin Books (South Africa) (Pty) Ltd, 24 Sturdee Avenue,
Rosebank, Johannesburg 2196, South Africa

Penguin Books Ltd, Registered Offices: 80 Strand, London WC2R 0RL, England

First published in 2007 by Viking Studio, a member of Penguin Group (USA) Inc.

10 9 8 7 6 5 4 3 2

Copyright © Melissa Pasanen and Shelburne Farms, 2007
Food photographs © Susie Cushner, 2007
All rights reserved.

Portrait photographs by Jordan Silverman (www.jordansilverman.com)
Photographs on pages 1, 33, 53, 77, 103, 157,
183, 207, 233 and 255 by Marshall Webb
Food styling by Jee Levin
Prop styling by Michele Michael

ISBN 978-0-670-01835-2

This book is printed on recycled paper.

Printed in the United States of America
Set in ITC New Baskerville
Designed by Stephanie Tevonian

Without limiting the rights under copyright reserved above, no part of this publication may be reproduced, stored in or introduced into a retrieval system, or transmitted, in any form or by any means (electronic, mechanical, photocopying, recording or otherwise), without the prior written permission of both the copyright owner and the above publisher of this book.

The scanning, uploading, and distribution of this book via the Internet or via any other means without the permission of the publisher is illegal and punishable by law. Please purchase only authorized electronic editions and do not participate in or encourage electronic piracy of copyrightable materials. Your support of the author's rights is appreciated.

For Alex, Nikko, Miles, and Luke—
may you never lose your wonder in
the earth's gifts and always be thankful
for the hands that nurture your food

Contents

Foreword

One of my earliest memories of growing up on Shelburne Farms with my five siblings was the aroma of manure from our dad's overalls hanging in the garage. At that time, our parents were focused on re-creating a viable farm enterprise from our decrepit family estate. My father converted a former golf course on the property into pasture for milking cows and built an innovative dairy pole barn in 1952, the year I was born. I remember hot summer days in haylofts, bringing home puffball mushrooms from the fields or strings of perch caught off Orchard Point, and collecting tubs of shiny brown horse chestnuts in the fall. A great old apple tree near our house must have been there when the Nash family was farming the same plot of land before our great-grandparents came to town.

Farming has always been at the heart of Shelburne Farms. What began as a neighborhood of small farms in the 1800s evolved in the 1880s into an expansive private agricultural estate and model farm founded by my great-grandparents, Dr. William Seward Webb and Lila Osgood Vanderbilt Webb. Today it is a vibrant membership-supported and trustee-governed educational organization and National Historic Landmark with a singular mission: to cultivate a conservation ethic. All of our programs help kindle human connections to nature and agriculture and build a sense of place and community.

That is what this cookbook is about too. I don't consider myself a sophisticated food person, but I love eating from the garden and eating food in season, especially when I know who produced it, where the farm is, and what the farming practices are. For me, food is all about good health and connections to people and the land. I feel so grateful whenever I have the opportunity to sit with friends on the terrace at our Inn at Shelburne Farms, enjoying a farm-fresh meal and beautiful summer evening with the sun setting over the lake and the Adirondack Mountains.

In the late 1960s, however, the future of Shelburne Farms was in doubt. Although the environmental movement was beginning to take shape, the forces of suburbanization were also gathering steam across the country, including here in Chittenden County, Vermont. Shelburne Farms seemed likely to become a string of subdivisions. Our family ultimately decided on a different course, opting to pursue an innovative land use and conservation plan so that the property could serve as an agriculture-based educational and community resource.

Farming and food were still center stage when the Farm began a new era as a nonprofit environmental education center in 1972. Our first summer youth camps were centered around growing garden produce and selling it at the local farmers' market. In those early years we made land available for community gardens and renovated barn space for a canning center. That space has been occupied for many years now by O-Bread Bakery (the smell of fresh-baked bread fills our offices daily). A raw milk bottling business had transitioned into our signature farmhouse cheddar cheese operation by the early 1980s. Our grass-based dairy, market garden, and woodland operations continue a long agricultural tradition on this land. These farm enterprises, including the original family residence, Shelburne House, which was transformed in 1987 into The Inn at Shelburne Farms, now help support the Farm's programs in serving a widening audience of schoolchildren and educators from Vermont and around the world.

Through this cookbook we celebrate and appreciate the "Farm" in Shelburne Farms and a growing understanding of how integral healthy local food systems are to creating a sustainable future. We invite you to visit and learn more about Shelburne Farms and our programs and encourage you to discover and support the farmers and food artisans closest to you.

Alec Webb, president of Shelburne Farms

About the Recipes

This cookbook is structured a little differently from many others—and that says a lot about why and how we wrote it. Instead of grouping recipes by type of dish (soups, salads, main courses, etc.), we build each chapter around an ingredient, or group of ingredients, that represents a part of Vermont's food heritage: from the native Abenakis' wild fish and game, to the lamb that symbolizes Vermont's sheep-farming boom of the 1800s, to state icons like maple, milk, and apples, which have defined our agricultural landscape for more than a century.

As part of its mission to cultivate a conservation ethic, Shelburne Farms is a dedicated supporter of local agriculture and is itself a creator of sustainably produced food. *Cooking with Shelburne Farms* is, in turn, a celebration of Vermont-grown food, and also of the farmers, cheesemakers, foragers, hunters and fishermen, and maple sugarmakers who cultivate, harvest, or craft it. It seemed only natural to let them and their ingredients lead the way.

Within these pages you will find over one hundred recipes inspired by nine ingredients and created to deliver a taste of Vermont in a fresh, comfortable, country-style cooking approach. There are recipes for low-fuss weeknight dinners—maple and black pepper roast chicken and crispy pork chops with green herb sauce—as well as dishes that will impress guests, such as roast duck legs with sour cherry sauce and smoke-grilled leg of lamb with eggplant and tomato salad. There are New England classics like hot milk sponge cake and apple pie, along with twists on hash, shepherd's pie, and tomato soup. We also pair native ingredients with newer world flavors, such as crushed fennel seed and orange zest rubbed onto a slow-roasted pork shoulder and venison chili with deep, spicy echoes of Mexican mole.

While the ingredients and recipes are grounded in Vermont, there are variation suggestions to encourage those of you in other parts of the country to make similar connections in your communities and develop your own sense of place through the food you cook and eat.

As you read about the sweet, smoky scent of a steaming sugarhouse, the anticipation of lambing, the treasure hunt for the first wild green shoots or prized mushrooms of the season, we hope you are inspired to think about where your food comes from and to treasure it and the land and people who bring it to you.

Melissa Pasanen and Chef Rick Gencarelli,
Shelburne Farms

Some General Guidelines to Our Recipes

Here are some basics that we don't spell out in each recipe. If the recipe calls for something different from the below, we will specify.

Equipment and Technique

- Pans are not nonstick.
- The oven rack is in the standard center position.
- When using the microwave, make sure to use a microwave-safe bowl.
- Oil is hot when it thins out and moves freely in the pan. This is the point you want to reach with most recipes to start softening onions or shallots. In another minute or two it will shimmer, the temperature you want for searing meat or mushrooms. A step further takes the pan to just about smoking, which you want only for very quick cooking tasks like searing scallops.
- *Deglaze* means to add liquid to a pan you have used to sauté something, bring the liquid to a simmer, and stir to scrape up any brown bits stuck to the pan and incorporate them into the liquid.
- When we specify instant-read thermometer temperatures, they are almost always a few degrees below the final desired temperature to account for carryover cooking during meat resting time.

Ingredients

- We almost always include a base level of salt in a dish and then encourage you to taste as you go and to adjust seasoning to your preference. We use coarse kosher salt when cooking and regular fine table salt when baking. They are not interchangeable: a teaspoon of coarse salt is less salt than the equivalent volume measurement of fine salt.
- Dairy products such as milk, buttermilk, yogurt, or sour cream can be any percent fat.
- Maple syrup can be any grade.
- Olive oil does not need to be extra virgin.
- Additional oil, butter, or flour for preparing pans is not included in the ingredients list.
- Cheddar is grated on the coarse holes of a box grater, and Parmesan is grated on the small holes of a box grater or rotary grater.
- Onions are yellow, and all onions, shallots, and garlic are peeled before using.
- If we don't specify a volume equivalent for a number of shallots or garlic, a little variation won't make any difference to the recipe result.

- Citrus zest is grated very finely with a rasp grater, such as a Microplane. Always take care to avoid the bitter white pith. As a general rule, if you're trying to figure out how many citrus fruits to buy to yield a specified amount of zest or juice:
  - 1 medium orange yields about 1 tablespoon finely grated zest and ⅓–½ cup juice.
  - 1 large lemon yields about 2–3 teaspoons finely grated zest and 2–3 tablespoons juice.
  - 1 medium lime yields about 2 teaspoons finely grated zest and 1–2 tablespoons juice.
- In cases where finished recipes contain raw or lightly cooked eggs, you may want to avoid serving those to young children, pregnant women, or anyone with compromised immune systems who are at increased risk of serious illness from any egg-borne *Salmonella enteritidis*.

Savory
Milk
and
Cheese

*e*very day throughout summer and fall in the Children's Farmyard at Shelburne Farms, a caramel-colored cow with soft, patient, dark eyes allows visiting children to try out their new milking skills. They learn to make a circle with their fingers and pull down gently but firmly on a warm teat. The first squirt of milk never fails to elicit surprise and delight.

Milk is our first food; it symbolizes purity and nurturing. Few raw ingredients are as versatile. It has infinite uses and forms: butter, cream, buttermilk, yogurt, cheeses—fresh and aged. Milk is often taken for granted even though it is at the core of many recipes. It is rarely the headline ingredient, more often working quietly in the background to bind, moisten, or enrich.

Dairy has been Vermont's most important agricultural product for more than 150 years, although the state's dairy farmers struggle today in a commodity market in which larger farms have advantages over typically smaller-scale Vermont agriculture. Many are going organic or creating local milk brands to keep small family farms alive and preserve the pastoral landscape dotted with red barns and grazing animals. A vibrant community of farmstead cheesemakers has built a reputation across the country for award-winning cheeses from the milk of their own cows, sheep, goats, and even water buffalo.

There has been a milking herd on Shelburne Farms without

interruption since 1889. During the era of founders Seward and Lila Webb, fresh milk, cream, and butter from Jersey, Holstein, and Durham cows were sent daily from the Southern Acres Dairy Barn to Shelburne House for the family and their guests, as well as shared with some employees. Dairy products were also shipped to various Webb residences and sold to the family's railroad businesses for use in the dining cars.

The origins of the current Brown Swiss pasture-raised herd go back to Derick Webb, Seward and Lila's grandson, who first recognized the strength of the breed in 1947 when he noted that a cross between Brown Swiss and Holstein was particularly good for dairy, "really milking fools." He later focused on a purely Brown Swiss herd, which he moved into a newly constructed pole-style dairy barn in 1952. The new barn sat in the middle of rich pastureland where the cows could graze, rather than be confined inside eating grain.

In 1979, the Webbs began selling natural raw milk to local markets under the Shelburne Farms label, but they soon decided that making cheese would be a better way to develop a steady income in support of their educational mission. Bill Clapp, who had been running the milk business, took on the cheesemaking with the assistance of one of Derick's sons, Marshall. The first batches, Bill admits with a chuckle, "were inedible, so acid that we threw them in

the compost and months later they still hadn't broken down."
Clapp took a trip to England to visit the famous Montgomery
cheddar estate. While there, he unexpectedly discovered his own
ancestral cheddar heritage and brought back a family recipe upon
which he based Shelburne Farms' ultimately award-winning cheese.

Home-Churned Butter

[photograph 1]

Shaking cream into butter is one of the most vivid memories many visitors—young and old—take away from the Shelburne Farms Children's Farmyard. Cream is poured into a small container and everyone takes a turn to shake it into sweet, fresh butter, singing as it makes its way around the circle. Food "manufacturing" was never so immediate, so personal, and so delicious. ◇ **Makes: About ⅓ cup**

1 cup heavy cream, at room temperature or, ideally, left out overnight

Table salt or coarse kosher salt to taste

Before You Start If you can find pasteurized cream (instead of ultrapasteurized), the butter will taste better and "churn" quicker. Leaving the cream out overnight to ripen just a touch also improves flavor and speeds up butter making and should not be cause for health concerns. You can make the butter in larger quantities (and containers) than detailed below; it will just take longer.

1. Select a small plastic container with a tight lid. (Little snack-size containers about 1½ inches square work well.) Fill it halfway with the cream and add a clean marble or pebble. You may want to wrap the container with a dish towel because aggressive shaking can cause leaks. (Don't use glass jars, which work well until a marble cracks them.)

2. Shake vigorously until you get butter, about 5–10 minutes depending on the size of the container, the temperature of the cream, and the persistence of the shaking.

3. Listen for the marble—at first, it sounds loud, then it becomes muffled for a while when the cream reaches a whipped stage, and then it gets loud again when the butter separates from the liquid.

4. When you have reached solid butter, pour off the buttermilk (to taste later), take out the marble, and add a little salt if you like. Repeat with the remaining cream.

From the Archives: In 1889, the *Albany Journal* noted that demand for "butter from Dr. Webb's famous farm" exceeded supply and that "prominent caterers have offered double prices for all that they could obtain." At its peak, the Shelburne Farms creamery made up to four hundred pounds of butter a week in two-pound molds with the impression of a sheaf of wheat. If the farm were to market butter today, it might bear the imprint of a red clover, the Vermont state flower and part of the pasture mix of plants the cows graze on.

Compound Butters

[photograph 1]

Fresh butter doesn't need much improvement, but with the addition of a few well-chosen flavorings, compound butters can dress up a plain piece of meat, take a vegetable from everyday to elegant, or add a touch of class to a breakfast tray. A few different flavors stored in the freezer are like money in the bank.

Start with ½ cup (8 tablespoons) of best-quality unsalted butter or homemade freshly churned butter at room temperature. Use a spoon or small spatula to work in the flavoring ingredients until thoroughly blended. Season to taste with salt if appropriate, and then either put the butter in a small serving bowl or roll it in wax paper to make a tube from which you can slice off disks. Well-sealed compound butter will keep in the refrigerator for up to a week and in the freezer for several months.

- For meat or fish steaks or fillets, set a chilled disk or spoonful of compound butter on the warm meat or fish as it rests after cooking.
- Place disks under the skin of chicken or in the middle of burger patties before cooking.
- Add a dollop to the hot broth of steamed shellfish right before serving.
- To make a quick pan sauce for meat, fish, or pasta, whisk compound butter by the tablespoonful into half a cup of hot pasta water, stock, or wine (off the flame) until the desired consistency is achieved.

Butter	Work in	Use on
Blue cheese–black pepper	2 tablespoons blue cheese 2 teaspoons freshly ground black pepper	beef, venison, burgers, pork, chicken, pasta, green beans, baked potatoes
Caper-parsley	2 tablespoons drained and coarsely chopped capers 1 tablespoon chopped flat-leaf parsley 1 teaspoon lemon juice ¼ teaspoon anchovy paste or ½ anchovy, finely minced	fish, chicken, steamed shellfish, cauliflower
Goat cheese	¼ cup soft fresh goat cheese at room temperature	chicken, sweet potatoes, winter squash, pasta, vegetables such as peas, green beans, broccoli
Honey-sage	2 tablespoons honey 1 tablespoon finely minced sage	chicken, duck, pork, delicate white fish such as trout or tilapia, breakfast muffins or tea scones
Horseradish	2 tablespoons prepared horseradish	beef, burgers, crab cakes, baked potatoes, salmon, ham
Mint-lemon	1 tablespoon finely chopped fresh mint 2 teaspoons finely grated lemon zest 1 teaspoon freshly squeezed lemon juice	lamb, white fish, chicken, vegetables such as asparagus, summer squash, peas, green beans
Mustard	1 tablespoon whole-grain mustard	beef, burgers, salmon, pork, chicken, meaty white fish like cod or halibut, green beans

Butter	Work in	Use on
Orange-rosemary	2 tablespoons orange marmalade 2 teaspoons finely chopped rosemary	pork, duck, breakfast muffins or tea scones
Peach-sage	2 tablespoons peach or apricot jam 2 teaspoons finely chopped sage	ham, pork, breakfast muffins or tea scones
Red wine–shallot	2 cups full-bodied red wine ¼ cup chopped shallots 1 bay leaf 6 black peppercorns 2 sprigs thyme (Bring to a boil and simmer until reduced to 2 tablespoons. Strain and cool before adding to butter.)	beef, venison, burgers, pork, chicken, salmon
Roasted scallion	4 scallions, grilled or roasted until slightly charred, then finely chopped 1 teaspoon finely grated lemon zest 1 teaspoon freshly squeezed lemon juice	seafood, chicken, burgers, green beans, peas, baked potatoes
Strawberry-tarragon	2 tablespoons strawberry jam 2 teaspoons finely chopped tarragon	breakfast muffins or tea scones

Smoked Cheddar Crackers

This melt-in-your-mouth cracker recipe is based on an old New England classic sometimes called "cheddar pennies." They are addictive when made with regular cheddar and even better made with Shelburne Farms' award-winning smoked cheddar and a dash of cayenne pepper. Shelburne Farms sends its cheddar to the monks of New Skete in rural upstate New York for a slow, old-fashioned smoke over hickory wood. These make a great party snack, cocktail nibble, or gift.

◇ ***Makes: About 80 bite-size crackers***

1½ cups all-purpose flour

1 teaspoon baking powder

½ teaspoon table salt

¼ teaspoon cayenne pepper

½ cup (1 stick) unsalted butter cut into 8 pieces, at room temperature

2 lightly packed cups (about 6 ounces) grated smoked cheddar (see Before You Start)

2–3 tablespoons buttermilk or plain yogurt (see Tip, page 12)

Before You Start You will want to use a best-quality smoked cheddar for this—one that is truly smoked and not made with artificial smoke flavor. If you can't find any, opt for a best-quality six-month to one-year aged cheddar or a best-quality smoked Gouda. If you don't have a food processor, you can mix this using an electric mixer, either standing or handheld. Cream the butter first, and then mix in the cheese, followed by the dry ingredients, which you have previously whisked together. Last, mix in the liquid just until the dough holds together.

1. In the bowl of a food processor fitted with the metal blade, pulse together the flour, baking powder, salt, and cayenne pepper.

2. Add the butter and pulse about ten times until the mixture is sandy. Add the grated cheese and pulse another five times until the mixture is pebbly.

3. With the food processor running, drizzle buttermilk through the feed tube just until the dough holds together.

4. On a lightly floured work surface, divide the dough into two balls. Roll each out into a log about 8 inches long and 1½ inches in diameter. Wrap in plastic or wax paper and chill in the refrigerator for at least 30 minutes and up to 1 hour. While the dough is chilling, preheat the oven to 400°F.

5. Unwrap the chilled dough and slice it into ¼-inch rounds. Arrange on ungreased cookie sheets and bake for 6–8 minutes, until golden brown. Cool completely before storing in an airtight container.

Tip: You can make your own buttermilk by stirring 1 tablespoon of white vinegar or lemon juice into 1 cup of milk and letting it sit for a few minutes to curdle. This soured milk works fine instead of buttermilk in most baking recipes but is not usually a good substitute in recipes that are not cooked, like dressings or cool soups. See page 25 for more tips on how to use buttermilk.

Prepare-Ahead Tip: You can freeze logs of dough for later use; just thaw them in the refrigerator overnight before baking.

Toasted Corn and Milk Chowder

Chowder is usually heavy with potatoes and cream; this lighter version delivers richness through summer-sweet corn pureed in milk. The smoked trout is not absolutely necessary, but it adds a great layer of flavor to the "chowdah," as we say here in New England. ◇ **Makes: 4 bowls or 6 cups**

2 tablespoons unsalted butter

2 small leeks (about ¾ pound), white and light green parts only, halved lengthwise, thinly sliced, and rinsed thoroughly

1½ cups corn kernels, from 2–3 ears corn (see Tip, page 14) or canned or frozen corn (see Before You Start)

1 teaspoon finely chopped fresh thyme leaves or ¼ teaspoon dried thyme

3 cups whole or 2 percent milk

1 teaspoon coarse kosher salt plus more to taste

3–4 ounces smoked trout, peeled from the skin and flaked

Freshly ground black pepper to taste

Before You Start Fresh corn is best for this recipe, but we found that canned or thawed frozen corn kernels worked fine as long as they were carefully patted dry with paper towel. You will find smoked trout near the smoked salmon at good fish counters.

1. In a large, wide soup pot, melt the butter over medium-high heat until foamy. Lower the heat to medium, add the leeks to the pot, and cook, stirring occasionally, until soft, about 5 minutes.

2. Add the corn and thyme and increase the heat to medium-high. Cook, stirring occasionally, until the corn is a toasty golden brown, another 7–9 minutes. Scoop out half the corn and leek mixture and set aside in a bowl.

3. Reduce the heat to medium and add 2 cups of the milk and the salt to the corn and leeks in the pot. Bring to a simmer and cook for 3–4 minutes.

4. Carefully pour the corn and milk mixture into a blender or food processor and puree until smooth. (Always use caution when blending hot liquids—see the Tip on page 14.) Pour the blended mixture through a fine-meshed sieve back into the pot, pressing on the solids to extract the smooth pulp and as much liquid as possible.

5. Over medium heat, stir in the remaining cup of milk and bring the chowder to a simmer. Return the reserved corn and leeks to the soup along with the trout. Heat through and adjust seasoning to taste. Serve immediately or chill and serve cool.

Tip: To cut corn from the cob without losing half the kernels as they fly all over the kitchen, lay a clean dish towel on your counter and stand the cob flat on its trimmed stalk end in the middle of the towel. With the sharpest knife you have, cut the kernels off from top to bottom, and you will find most will fall within the range of the towel. Just pick the towel up and dump all the kernels into the pot.

Tip: Use great care with the food processor or blender when blending hot liquids like soups. If you put the lid on tightly, steam can build up. Leave the center of the blender lid off or the feed tube of the food processor open, and cover the opening with a wadded dish towel. Start blending slowly, and don't overfill the machine; blend in batches if necessary.

Tomato-Cheddar Soup

A steaming bowl of cream of tomato soup is always wonderful paired with a gooey grilled cheese sandwich. We decided to put the soup and the cheddar all in one bowl, making for a familiar yet unexpected taste. If you really want to go all the way, melt a little more grated cheddar on a piece of toasted crusty bread and set it adrift in your soup. ◇ **Makes: 4 bowls or 6 cups**

1 packed cup (about 4 ounces) finely grated cheddar

1 tablespoon all-purpose flour

2 tablespoons unsalted butter

1 small onion, diced (about ⅓ cup)

1 cup half-and-half or whole milk

1 (28-ounce) can whole tomatoes in puree, preferably fire-roasted (see Before You Start)

1 teaspoon ground allspice

½ teaspoon coarse kosher salt plus more to taste

Freshly ground black pepper to taste

Before You Start   Buy the best sharp cheddar you can find, aged six months to one year. Once you add the cheese to the soup, it is important not to let it boil. If you cannot find canned, fire-roasted tomatoes such as those made by Muir Glen, buy whole canned tomatoes, drain them (reserving their puree), lay them on a rimmed cookie sheet and put them under a hot broiler for about 3–4 minutes per side until lightly charred. Then use them with the reserved puree as directed in step 6.

1. In a small bowl, toss the grated cheddar with the flour, making sure to coat all shreds. Set aside.

2. In a large, wide soup pot set over medium-high heat, melt the butter until foamy. Add the onion and cook, stirring occasionally, until translucent but not colored, about 3–4 minutes.

3. Add the half-and-half to the pot, bring to a simmer, and simmer gently for 3–4 minutes. Take the pot off the heat.

4. Using your hands, lift the cheddar from the bowl and whisk handfuls into the hot half-and-half mixture until the mixture is smooth.

5. Add the tomatoes with their puree, the allspice, and the salt to the soup base and stir. Return the pot to medium heat for 3–4 minutes and cook, stirring to blend. Do not allow the soup to boil.

6. Using an immersion blender, a food processor, or a blender, blend the soup in batches. (Always use caution blending hot liquids—see the Tip on page 14.)

7. Return the soup to the pot over medium-low heat and warm it gently just until a few bubbles rise to the surface. Adjust seasoning to taste and serve.

Watermelon, Tomato, and Feta Salad

[photograph 2]

The combination of watermelon and tomatoes might have raised eyebrows a few years ago, but then chefs realized that August could not pass without pairing two of the month's all-stars. Rick's version at the Inn—which he first learned from his mentor, Todd English at Olives—is served in a chilled bowl with all ingredients chilled except the tomatoes. It is the perfect antidote to a steamy hot day.

◇ *Serves: 4*

1 large red tomato (about ½ pound), cored and chunked

12 large fresh mint leaves, coarsely chopped, plus a few more whole leaves for garnish

1½ cups bite-size cubes seeded watermelon

2 large tomatoes (about 1 pound), any color, cored and cut into bite-size cubes, or about ¾ pound cherry or pear tomatoes in assorted colors, sliced in half

1½ teaspoons coarse kosher salt

Freshly ground black pepper to taste

2 teaspoons extra-virgin olive oil

2 teaspoons champagne vinegar or white wine vinegar

½ cup (about 2–3 ounces) crumbled feta

Before You Start The different shades of red from the watermelon and tomatoes make this gorgeous, but it's also fun to mix colors by finding yellow watermelon or, alternatively, yellow pear tomatoes or small orange cherry tomatoes. It is worth searching out fresh, locally made feta for this salad—in Vermont we like the goat version from Does' Leap Farm in East Fairfield and Bonnieview Farm's sheep milk feta made in Craftsbury Common (see Sources, page 273). It goes without saying that the salad is not worth making with lackluster, off-season tomatoes.

1. Put the chunked tomato into a blender and puree until completely smooth. Set a fine sieve over a medium bowl, pour the tomato puree into the sieve, and allow to drain for at least 10 minutes. Reserve the resulting tomato water, which should be about ¼–⅓ cup.

2. In another medium bowl, combine the chopped mint, watermelon, tomato cubes, salt, a few grinds of pepper, the olive oil, and the champagne vinegar. Toss gently to combine.

3. Prepare salads individually by spooning a tablespoon of the reserved tomato water onto a plate (chilled if you like), topping it with a quarter of the watermelon and tomato mixture, sprinkling 2 tablespoons of crumbled feta on top, and garnishing with a mint leaf. Serve immediately.

Following the Milk

Sam Dixon, dairy farmer, and Jaime Yturriondobeitia, cheesemaker, Shelburne Farms

"Farming's about stewardship and husbandry, taking care of the land and taking care of the animals."

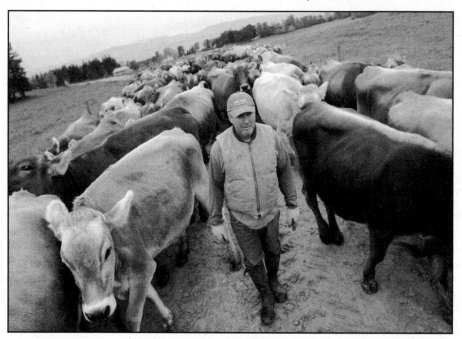

S tars are often still in the sky when Shelburne Farms dairy farmer Sam Dixon fetches the cows from the fields for the morning milking. As the 115 Brown Swiss make their steady approach, guided by the glow from the milking parlor, Sam walks along, opening gates and making sure stragglers keep up. At four thirty, the birds haven't started singing yet; there are only quiet hoofsteps and a few soft lows. One cow stops and nuzzles Sam like a dog. "Some like to be petted," he says as he rubs her head.

Milking is the start of each day and the foundation of the Farm's cheddar cheese. "If the milk's not good, the cheese is not good," says cheesemaker Jaime Yturriondobeitia.

Before there can be milk, there must be sun and rain to nurture the grass and other pasture plants. During the growing season, the herd feeds largely on pasture, rotating into a new field every twelve to twenty-four hours to take optimal advantage of the nutrition in each paddock and to allow the plants a chance to grow back between grazings. Because grass-based dairy farming closely follows natural cycles, many believe it is the most environmentally responsible way to raise healthy animals. "Farming's about stewardship and husbandry," Sam emphasizes, "taking care of the land and taking care of the animals."

While the cows are being milked, Sam feeds the calves, who look up at him with huge, heavy-lashed eyes as he pours milk into their feed buckets. He stops to bottle-feed a silver-gray bull calf born just a few days earlier. The calf bucks a little at the slightly chilly milk, but Sam gently persists. He grew up on a small homestead farm in southern Vermont where his family hand-milked their cow and raised a litter of piglets each year. "Farming has always been what I wanted to do," Sam reflects. "I would die if I had to go sit in a cubicle in front of a computer."

It's getting tougher to find the next generation of farmers, he says. "It's hard work, the hours are long, and it's dirty," and, for the most part, he continues, "our society doesn't put a lot of value on the labor or the knowledge, like how to treat cows and work with them." But there are rewards too, Sam adds. "The other night, driving down after putting the cows out, it was so beautiful and the pastures were so green," he recalls. "It was a tough summer, but the collective work of the crew got us through."

. . . .

"If the milk's not good, the cheese is not good."

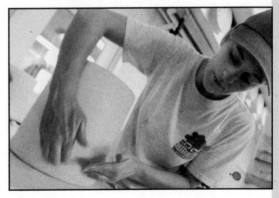

*t*he day has dawned by the time a member of the cheesemaking team arrives to drive the milk down to the 120-year-old Farm Barn. The driver holds a scribbled note of the milk weight up against the window of the cheesemaking room before turning the spigot to allow the fresh milk to bubble and eddy into the open vat. Small floating islands of golden fat appear in a few places, and Jaime explains that the butterfat ratio is very high in late-season milk like today's and that the short road trip has jostled the fat molecules about, making them more likely to separate.

As the milk flows in, Jaime finishes taking yesterday's blocks of cheddar out of the molds in which they were pressed overnight. She extracts a few long plugs of cheese for testing. If you took a bite now, she says, it would taste "oaty, grassy—like if you pick a blade of grass with seeds and chew on it." Each batch will vary slightly, she clarifies. "I taste a lot of cheese, and every day it's different."

While the milk heats, Jaime works on the tall cylinders of cheese destined to become Shelburne Farms clothbound cheddar. She shaves their surface smooth with a knife and wraps lard-soaked muslin tightly around each one, meticulously flattening any air bubbles.

About two hours after the milk arrives, the cheesemakers add rennet to the vat. "This is my favorite part of the day," Jaime says. You can actually see the milk gel into a solid, she explains, showing how she tests it with a knife and with her finger to see when a break in the developing curd seals cleanly. Another way she checks is to lightly place her palm on the soft, warm surface to see if an impression remains when she pulls her hand away. "I like it because it feels alive," she says.

The room fills with a sweet, milky aroma as the whey drains from the vat into a holding tank. Most of it will be spread over the fields, coming full circle. "Some days it smells so good, like cream," says Jaime. "You just want to add strawberries and jump right in."

If you ask Bill Clapp—the first cheesemaker at the Farm back in 1980—what is the most critical factor in making Shelburne Farms cheddar, he answers, "Brown Swiss cows and raw milk, right off the bat. That is the best milk. You cannot miss making a great cheese with milk of that quality. I never bought milk. Always just went to the bulk tank. I still miss it."

Green Mountain Ploughman's Lunch and Picnic Tips

[photograph 3]

The ploughman's lunch is a British tradition, the meal classically taken by farm workers to the fields and a pub favorite. It usually consists of good crusty bread or rolls, a hunk of farmhouse cheddar or other locally made firm cheese, tangy Branston Pickle chutney, and bite-size pickled onions.

For a Green Mountain version, start with a loaf of naturally leavened bread like the French batard or sesame wheat bread from O-Bread, the European-style bakery that has baked up wonderful aromas and bread in the Shelburne Farms Farm Barn since 1977. Add a good hunk of Shelburne Farms cheddar—perhaps the three-year, with its pleasing dry, crumbly texture and nutty bite. Pack up a small jar of our Apple-Rhubarb Chutney (page 215) and some Pickled Ramps (page 59) made with the aromatic wild leeks that are abundant during springtime in Vermont. Finish with a few crisp apples.

Shelburne Farms is full of perfect spots where you can enjoy your ploughman's—from the lawn behind the Inn, where thousands picnic every summer during Vermont Mozart Festival concerts, to the top of Lone Tree Hill, which "seems to me like heaven," as Lila Webb wrote in her 1922 Christmas greeting. But no matter where you are, there are always places that call out for a picnic. Here are a few hints to help you fit more spontaneous picnics into your life.

- **Be prepared**. Keep a basket of picnic supplies ready, including essentials like a blanket, small cutting board and sharp knife, trash bag, and bug repellent. A set of inexpensive plastic or tin plates, cutlery, napkins, and cups are nice to have too. If your picnic hardware is ready any time, then all you have to do is throw the food in the basket and you're off.
- **Keep it simple.** As in the ploughman's described above, good bread, cheese, fruit, and a cool drink make a great picnic. If you like, add some salami or cold roast chicken and a box of fancy cookies.
- **Create without cooking.** When it feels too warm to turn on the stove, turn to other kitchen tools to add something a little different without much work at all. Try whipping up a cold soup like the Cucumber-Yogurt Soup (page 22) in a blender, or use the food processor to make our Deviled Ham and Cheddar Spread (page 168).
- **Make it special** with a few flowers, candles in small jars, or bubbles for blowing.

Savory Milk and Cheese

Cucumber-Yogurt Soup

Add a touch of cool elegance to your picnic or summer meal with this easy blender soup. ◇ **Makes: 4 bowls or 6 cups**

2 long English cucumbers (about 1¼ pounds total), peeled and cut into chunks (see Before You Start)

½ cup chopped fresh cilantro leaves

2 cups plain yogurt

2 tablespoons olive oil

2 tablespoons freshly squeezed lime juice

1 teaspoon ground cumin

2 teaspoons coarse kosher salt plus more to taste

Buttermilk, milk, or water to thin soup as needed

Before You Start   If you can't find English cucumbers, use regular cucumbers, but after peeling them, slice them lengthwise down the middle and use a spoon to scoop out their watery seeds.

1. Place the cucumbers, cilantro, yogurt, olive oil, lime juice, cumin, and salt in a blender and puree until smooth. Thin with buttermilk if desired. Adjust seasoning to taste.

2. Serve at room temperature or chill before serving.

Prepare-Ahead Tip: *This is even better when made ahead. Bring it on a picnic in an insulated thermos.*

Cheese Plate Basics

In Vermont, we are lucky to have a rich array of small farmstead cheesemakers, and we look for every opportunity to taste and enjoy the diversity of cheese they create. A cheese tasting plate can take many forms and fit many venues. It's a great icebreaker for any party. Farmers' markets across the country are a wonderful way to meet and taste the work of small regional cheesemakers. (For more information on Vermont cheesemakers or to find small cheesemakers near you, see Sources, page 273.)

Here are some tips on how to put together a cheese plate:

- Three to five different cheeses is a good number for the average gathering. Estimate ½–1 ounce per person per cheese depending on what else is being offered and when you are presenting the cheeses.
- Select cheeses made from a variety of milks, such as cow, sheep, and goat, and in a variety of textures, from soft and spreadable to crumbly to firm. (Or pick cheeses all made from one type of milk but with contrasting textures and flavors.)
- Go for a variety of flavors from mild to strong, and arrange the tray in that order so that a strong blue cheese, for example, does not overwhelm more delicate cheeses.
- Buy cheese from a store that does a brisk business in cheese and, ideally, cuts cheese to order.
- Cheese needs to breathe. If your cheese comes wrapped in plastic, take the plastic off at home and rewrap the cheese in wax paper or parchment paper and then loosely in plastic wrap. Store cheese in your vegetable drawer or the most humid part of your refrigerator, and don't keep it too long.
- Bring all cheeses to room temperature before serving.
- Label each cheese so guests know what they're tasting; you can even take the labels off the cheeses and use those as tags.
- Add color to the plate with fresh or dried fruit, fruit preserves like Oven-Roasted Applesauce and Apple Butter (page 229) or Apple-Rhubarb Chutney (page 215), or some local honey. Fresh, raw vegetables like radishes, baby carrots, or slender green beans can also complement cheeses and clear the palate between tastes.
- Wine is fine, but many experts are now counseling that beer can be a better match for cheese, perhaps an India pale ale with an aged cheddar or a summer wheat beer with fresh chèvre. Hard cider is also a nice change.

Cheddar and Herb Biscuits

Nothing beats a good biscuit, especially if it is golden and fragrant with cheddar and fresh herbs. These are wonderful with soup, with stews, or as a topping for potpies like our Mushroom and Root Vegetable Potpie (page 120).
◇ *Makes: Twelve 2½-inch biscuits.*

3 cups all-purpose flour

2 tablespoons baking powder

½ teaspoon baking soda

1 teaspoon table salt

6 tablespoons cold unsalted butter, cut into small bits

1 cup (about 4 ounces) grated cheddar

2 tablespoons chopped fresh thyme, sage, or rosemary leaves

1¼ cups cold buttermilk plus a little more to brush the biscuit tops (see Tips, pages 12 and 25)

Before You Start Go for an aged sharp cheddar like one- or two-year Shelburne Farms. The key to light and flaky biscuits is to keep the ingredients as cold as possible and to work the dough as little as possible. Rick and I experienced proof of this when we mixed and rolled out multiple batches of biscuits in the unheated, off-season Inn kitchen in January. We were a little chilly, but the biscuits were perfect.

1. Preheat the oven to 425°F. In a large bowl, whisk together the flour, baking powder, baking soda, and salt.

2. With your fingers or two forks, work the butter into the flour mixture until the dough looks like fine gravel with a few larger butter bumps throughout. (Alternatively, use a food processor with a few short pulses.) Stir in the cheddar and thyme. Add the buttermilk gradually, just until a pinch of dough comes together when you squeeze it between your fingers.

3. Lightly flour the counter and dump the dough onto it. Knead it a few times to bring it together and then use a lightly floured rolling pin to roll the dough out ¾-inch thick. Cut out the biscuits with a 2½-inch cutter or a glass. (You can reroll scraps once but not more or the biscuits will be tough.)

4. Place the biscuits on an ungreased cookie sheet and brush the tops with buttermilk. Bake for 15–20 minutes, until golden brown.

> **Tip:** *We love buttermilk for its smooth, low-fat creaminess and the extra tang it brings to everything from soups to sherbet. If you buy a quart of buttermilk for a recipe that only calls for a cup or so, there are lots of good ways to put the extra to use. Try a cool soup like our Cucumber-Yogurt Soup (page 22) or a sherbet like our Buttermilk-Plum Sherbet (page 254). Buttermilk can be frozen in one-cup portions and thawed to use in baked goods like these biscuits. It can also be used in place of yogurt in pancake recipes like Apple and Cinnamon-Sugar Pancakes (page 212) for a slightly thinner batter. Or whisk up a quick, light buttermilk dressing by combining ¾ cup of buttermilk (preferably not nonfat), ¼ cup of sour cream, 1 tablespoon of freshly squeezed lemon juice, 1 teaspoon of coarse kosher salt, and ½ teaspoon of sugar. Adjust seasoning to taste and serve over everything from an iceberg wedge with crumbled blue cheese to cabbage slaw or our Beet, Apple, and Radish Salad (page 191). This dressing gets even better after a couple of days in the refrigerator.*

Cream-Roasted Fennel

This is a simple but luxurious way to convert nonbelievers to fennel, the lightly licorice-flavored vegetable that is sometimes called anise. It is all you need to perk up a dinner of plain roast or sautéed chicken, broiled fish, or pork chops.
◇ *Serves: 4*

1 large fennel bulb (about 1 pound with stalks)

3 tablespoons unsalted butter

1 tablespoon sugar

1 teaspoon coarse kosher salt

½ cup chicken stock, preferably low sodium

½ cup heavy cream

Before You Start Look for fennel bulbs that are plump and white. For this recipe, it is fine if the stalks with their feathery fronds have been cut off, although it is nice to sprinkle a few chopped fronds on the dish to serve. Be careful choosing your pan, as some ovenproof skillets are not up to the high heat of the broiler.

1. Trim the stalks from the fennel if they are still attached, reserving some fronds for garnish if desired. Set the root end down on a cutting board and cut the fennel down the middle lengthwise. Place one half of the fennel, cut side down, on the cutting board and cut ¼-inch-wide slices from the root to the stem. Repeat with the other half. The goal is that most pieces will still be held together by the root.

2. Preheat your broiler on its highest setting with a rack in the top slot.

3. In your largest broiler-proof sauté pan or skillet, melt the butter over medium-high heat until foamy. Add the fennel slices flat side down and sprinkle with the sugar and salt. (If they don't fit in one layer, you will need to do this in batches, adding a little more butter, sugar, and salt as necessary, and then put all the fennel back into the pan in two layers before adding the stock.) Cook until golden brown on one side, 5–7 minutes, without moving to ensure best caramelization. Then turn to the other side and cook until golden brown.

4. Add the stock to the pan and bring to a simmer. Cook 3–5 minutes, until the root end of the fennel gives easily to a fork.

5. Pour the cream over the fennel and put the pan under the broiler for 3–5 minutes until bubbly and brown in spots. Sprinkle with reserved, coarsely chopped fennel fronds as desired and serve immediately.

Variation This cream-roasting method works well for other sturdy vegetables such as leeks (white and light green parts only, halved lengthwise and rinsed thoroughly), brussels sprouts (small ones left whole and large ones cut in half through the root end), green cabbage (cored and cut into ½-inch-wide cross-section wedges), and cauliflower (prepared the same as the cabbage). Stovetop cooking times will vary. Cook until the thickest part of the vegetable gives easily to a fork.

Macaroni and Cheese with Ham and Horseradish

Macaroni and cheese is comfort food at its finest. This version distinguishes itself with a kick of horseradish, nicely browned nuggets of Vermont ham, and big, craggy croutons on top. Not to mention great cheddar cheese. ◇ **Serves: 8**

1 pound medium pasta shells

3 tablespoons olive oil

½ pound ham steak, diced into ¼-inch cubes (about 2 cups)

6 tablespoons unsalted butter

½ cup all-purpose flour

1 tablespoon horseradish or more to taste

4 cups milk

1 pound coarsely grated cheddar

20 chives, snipped with scissors into ½-inch lengths (about ⅓ cup)

Coarse kosher salt to taste

Freshly ground black pepper to taste

4–5 thick slices crusty, country-style bread, lightly toasted and chopped to make 2½ cups coarse crumbs

¼ cup freshly grated Parmesan

Before You Start The horseradish adds a nice little (really) kick. Fresh horseradish will add more heat, but the jarred kind will work well too. It will look like you have a lot of cheese sauce, but the macaroni will continue to drink it up as the dish bakes. A cheese sauce is best made with a younger, moister cheddar like Shelburne Farms six- or nine-month.

1. Preheat the oven to 350°F and lightly butter a 9 by 13-inch baking dish.

2. Put a large pot of salted water on to boil for the pasta. Cook according to package directions, just until al dente (or they still have a little resistance to the tooth). Drain the pasta and rinse with cold water to prevent sticking.

3. In a large, heavy-bottomed sauté pan or skillet set over medium-high heat, heat 1 tablespoon of the olive oil for 2–3 minutes. Add the ham and cook, stirring occasionally, until browned, about 5–7 minutes. Remove the ham from the pan and set aside.

4. Set the sauté pan back over medium heat, melt the butter until foamy, whisk in the flour, and cook, whisking constantly, 3–4 minutes, until the mixture turns a light tan color. Whisk in the horseradish.

5. Add the milk to the pan, whisking constantly, and bring the sauce to a simmer. Cook until the mixture is thick enough that a line drawn by your finger across a coated spoon leaves a mark, another 1–2 minutes. Take the pan off the heat and stir in the cheddar.

6. Pour the pasta into the pan of cheese sauce, add the ham and chives, and stir gently but thoroughly to combine. Adjust seasoning to taste and add more horseradish if desired. Pour the mixture into the prepared baking dish.

7. In a small bowl, combine the bread crumbs with the Parmesan and the remaining 2 tablespoons of olive oil. Spread evenly over the top of the macaroni.

8. Bake in the oven until the top is golden and bubbly, about 25–30 minutes.

Prepare-Ahead Tip: This dish can be prepared up to one day ahead, covered with a piece of foil (lightly oiled so the bread crumbs don't stick to it), and kept refrigerated. Increase the cooking time by 25 minutes and leave the foil on for the first 25 minutes.

Milk-Braised Chicken with Sage and Bay

This recipe was inspired by the classic Italian milk-braised pork, although we don't cook it nearly as long, making it a good weeknight dinner option. The milk makes a rich, lightly sweet sauce for the flavorful dark-meat chicken, while the sage and bay add a woodsy note—and a touch of history. A distinctive part of Lila Webb's original gardens behind Shelburne House was a row of large and perfectly manicured potted bay trees along the balustrade above Lake Champlain.

◇ *Serves: 4–6*

¼ cup all-purpose flour

1 teaspoon coarse kosher salt plus more to taste

½ teaspoon freshly ground black pepper plus more to taste

8–12 bone-in chicken thighs, about 3½–4 pounds (see Before You Start)

3 tablespoons olive oil

2 tablespoons chopped fresh sage (about 20 large leaves)

4 garlic cloves, thinly sliced

1 small onion, thinly sliced

1 cup dry white wine

3 bay leaves

1 cup whole milk

1–2 teaspoons freshly squeezed lemon juice

Before You Start   You can make this recipe with skin-on or skinless bone-in chicken thighs. The milk sauce will break and look curdled. This does not hurt the flavor, but if you don't like the way it looks after the dish is finished, pull the chicken off to a plate, remove the bay leaves, and quickly puree the sauce in a blender to reemulsify it. (Always use caution blending hot liquids—see the Tip on page 14.) Add the sauce back to the chicken and finish with the lemon juice as described below.

1. Preheat the oven to 375°F. In a wide, shallow, rimmed plate or bowl, stir together the flour, salt, and pepper. Pat the chicken dry and dredge it in the flour mixture.

2. In a large sauté pan or skillet (ideally large enough to fit all the chicken in one layer), heat the olive oil over medium-high heat until it is hot. Add the chicken to the pan (skin side down if you are using skin-on chicken) and cook, without moving, for 7–8 minutes until golden brown. Turn and repeat for the other side. Remove the chicken to a plate.

3. Drain all but 1 tablespoon of fat from the pan and discard. Put the pan back over medium-high heat and add the sage, garlic, and onion. Cook for 1–2 minutes, stirring, until the onion is softened. Add the wine and bay leaves and bring to a simmer, scraping up any brown bits. Simmer for 3–4 minutes.

4. Return the chicken and any accumulated juices to the pan. Add the milk and bring to a simmer. Cover with a lid or with foil and bake in the oven for 15 minutes. Remove the lid and bake for another 10 minutes, or until the chicken is cooked through and the sauce is somewhat reduced. (The chicken should register 175°F on an instant-read thermometer.)

5. Remove the bay leaves and stir in the lemon juice, starting with 1 teaspoon and adding more to taste. (Follow the directions in Before You Start on page 30 to puree the sauce if desired.) Adjust seasoning to taste and serve.

Savory Milk and Cheese

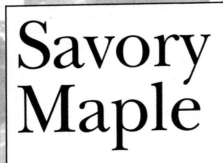

Savory
Maple

*i*f you get dripped on in a sugarhouse, it's good luck, they say. That's a good thing, because there's pretty much no way to spend time in a sugarhouse without being anointed with condensation from the sweet steam of the sap as it boils down into amber syrup. Of course, even without the drips, you are lucky to be there in the first place, drinking in the smoke-laced aroma, knowing that spring is finally on its way, and taking part in tradition.

The Shelburne Farms sugarhouse sits toward the bottom of Lone Tree Hill below a stand of sugar maples, what is known as a sugarbush. Around it, a web of tubing strung from tree to tree flows with sap each March, when warmer days alternate with chilly nights and the lifeblood of the trees starts to run. The clear liquid holds just a hint of the syrup's eventual deeply sweet flavor, achieved by hours of steady simmering in an evaporator over a wood-stoked fire until the ideal sugar content is reached. The finished syrup is drawn off, filtered into jugs, and sent over to the Inn.

Legends describe the discovery of the sweetness within the maple tree in various ways. The tale shared with visitors around the campfire next to the Shelburne Farms sugarhouse involves a native hunter who notched his tomahawk into a sugar maple for safe storage one night. When his children went to fetch water the next day, they left their empty pot at the foot of the tree while they ran off to play.

The pot mysteriously filled with clear liquid, and the venison their mother cooked in it had an unusually sweet flavor. The liquid, they discovered, was not water but sap dripping from the hatchet notch in the tree.

The first settlers learned from the natives to make "Indian molasses" or "Indian sugar," a homemade sweetener used when white sugar was rare and expensive. Although it can be hard to find today, maple sugar—then solidified into cakes—was the common form before refrigeration enabled longer-term storage of syrup. The Quakers promoted it as slave-free sugar, and Thomas Jefferson, who planted a sugarbush at Monticello, hoped that maple sugar might make the country more self-sufficient. Founded in 1893, the Vermont Maple Sugar Makers' Association claims to be the oldest agricultural association in the country, and the state is the largest U.S. producer of maple syrup.

Marshall Webb recalls backyard sugaring as a youngster, gathering sap the old-fashioned way and boiling it down over a fire until it could be finished off on the stove. "It would take us a couple of weeks to make a few quarts," he chuckles. His father, Lila and Seward Webb's grandson Derick, installed an evaporator in the Coach Barn, and the project expanded to include the sap from 150 buckets hung in a stand of sugar maples near the Market Garden. When education programs started in the Coach Barn, a small sugarhouse was built nearby, and a larger one was erected behind the Farm Barn a few years after it opened to the public in 1993. Sugaring on the Farm is largely an educational enterprise and the syrup is used for cooking at the Inn.

A Note on Maple
Grades

Vermont has four grades of retail maple syrup:

- Vermont Fancy is light-colored and delicately flavored. Its lighter flavor may get lost in cooking, but it is perfect on top of pancakes or ice cream.
- Grade A Medium Amber is slightly darker in color and deeper in flavor and works well for cooking and eating straight.
- Grade A Dark Amber is another step darker and deeper and is probably the preferred syrup of most sugarmakers for all-around use.
- Grade B is the darkest and strongest syrup available to consumers. It is a very good—and most economical—choice for cooking, as the maple flavor really comes through.

Other states and maple-producing regions have slightly different names—and criteria—for their grades. The New York equivalent of Vermont Grade B, for example, is "extra dark for cooking."

Granulated maple sugar is also sold regionally and in some natural foods markets. See Sources, page 273. Its texture and behavior in cooking are similar to granulated white sugar, although its flavor is more like brown sugar. It can sometimes benefit from a whir in the food processor to even out its texture.

Use and Storage Tips

- We usually cook with Grade A Dark Amber and bake with Grade B. Throughout this book, we specify if we recommend one over the other.
- Keep your maple syrup in the refrigerator or in the freezer, where it will thicken but not freeze.
- Try to remember to wipe off the rim of the container with a damp paper towel before closing it after each use. You will thank yourself the next time you want to open it.
- When measuring maple syrup, lightly oil the measuring cup so that it slips out easily. (This works for honey too.)

- Maple syrup can often substitute for brown sugar, molasses, or honey. When replacing molasses or honey, it can usually be used without other recipe changes. If substituting maple syrup for any type of sugar, you can trade them roughly cup for cup, but understand the following:
  - o Baking recipes are a lot more sensitive and will require a little experimentation. You may have to decrease other liquids by as much as ¼ cup.
  - o If you are baking and the recipe does not already call for it, you will need to add a little baking soda (¼ teaspoon will usually do it) to balance the acidity of the maple syrup.
  - o Recipes made with maple syrup will brown more quickly, so watch temperature carefully, decreasing if necessary or covering your food with foil to prevent overbrowning.
  - o Do not even think about using "table" or "pancake" syrup in place of pure maple syrup. It will not yield the same results and is a crime against nature.

Inn at Shelburne Farms Maple-Ginger Vinaigrette

This has been a fixture at the Inn since the restaurant's first chef, David Taylor, created it back in 1987, and it has many uses beyond salad as a marinade or pan sauce. ◇ ***Makes: 1½ cups***

1 medium clove garlic

1 medium shallot

1-inch piece fresh ginger root, peeled and coarsely chopped

2 tablespoons Dijon mustard

2 tablespoons soy sauce

2 tablespoons pure maple syrup

3 tablespoons balsamic vinegar

½ cup olive oil

½ cup canola oil

Coarse kosher salt to taste

Freshly ground black pepper to taste

1. In a blender or food processor, combine the garlic, shallot, ginger, mustard, soy sauce, maple syrup, and balsamic vinegar until well blended.

2. With the motor running on low, pour the olive and canola oils gradually through the hole in the blender lid or food processor feed tube and blend until emulsified.

3. Adjust seasoning to taste. Strain if desired.

Variation To marinate salmon, pork, or beef such as flank, hanger, or skirt steak with this vinaigrette, use about 2 tablespoons of vinaigrette per 8-ounce piece of fish or meat and marinate for 3–4 hours in the refrigerator before cooking. You can also use it as a glaze or quick pan sauce for scallops or shrimp, reducing it in the pan first. Avoid long, high-heat cooking because the maple syrup can burn.

Prepare-Ahead Tip: *The vinaigrette can be made two or three days ahead of time and kept refrigerated.*

Spiced Maple Nuts

These are wonderful as holiday gifts or cheese platter nibbles, or coarsely chopped on top of salads. They offer a medium kick—amp up the paprika and cayenne if you like more heat. (Or skip the spice coating and you'll just have nice, sweet, glazed nuts.) ◇ **Makes: 2 cups**

For the spice coating

1 teaspoon coarse kosher salt

1 teaspoon sweet or smoked sweet paprika

¼ teaspoon finely ground black pepper

¼ teaspoon cayenne pepper

2 teaspoons granulated maple sugar (see A Note on Maple, page 38) or light brown sugar

For the nuts

2 tablespoons unsalted butter

½ cup pure maple syrup

½ teaspoon coarse kosher salt

2 cups pecan halves

Before You Start If you can find smoked Spanish paprika (see Sources, page 273), it adds a nice smoky note to the nuts. You can use pretty much any nut you like—walnuts, cashews, almonds, or hazelnuts. The key to this simple recipe is getting the maple syrup hot enough, but not too hot, and then working very quickly to coat the nuts and spread them out before the syrup hardens. Practice or a candy thermometer are two avenues to success.

1. ***Make the spice coating:*** In a large bowl, whisk together the salt, paprika, black pepper, cayenne pepper, and maple sugar. Set aside.

2. ***Make the nuts:*** Lightly grease a cookie sheet or lay a nonstick baking mat on a cookie sheet or flat surface where it can remain undisturbed while the nuts cool.

3. In a medium, heavy-bottomed saucepan, melt the butter with the maple syrup and salt over medium-high heat. Bring to a boil and boil for about 10 minutes. The syrup should foam and become very dark brown. If you have a candy thermometer, you want the syrup to reach 290°F.

4. Take the pan off the heat and immediately stir in the pecans, coating them well with the syrup. Quickly pour the hot pecans into the bowl with the spice mixture and stir to coat the nuts evenly.

5. Dump the coated nuts onto the prepared cookie sheet and spread them out to cool. Cool the nuts completely and break them apart as desired.

Variation Try a similar method with butternut squash seeds or pepitas (hulled pumpkin seeds) to make Maple-Glazed Squash Seeds, a salty-sweet, crunchy garnish for the Maple-Roasted Butternut Squash Puree or Soup (page 202), or just for snacking. Toss the well-dried seeds of one squash (⅓–½ cup of seeds) with 2 teaspoons of olive oil and 1 teaspoon of coarse kosher salt and toast until golden. Boil ⅓ cup maple syrup for 3 minutes, stir in the toasted squash seeds, and boil, stirring, for another 3 minutes. Scoop out and cool as described above.   *[photograph 17]*

Red Cabbage, Pear, and Cranberry Slaw with Maple-Yogurt Dressing

We loved how all these flavors and textures worked together so much that we experimented with the combination both cool and warm and ended up with both a slaw and a braise (page 46). This slaw makes a great side for our Maple-Glazed Ribs (page 171). ◇ *Serves: 6*

1 small shallot, minced

½ cup pure maple syrup

2 tablespoons cider vinegar

½ cup plain yogurt

1½ teaspoons coarse kosher salt plus more to taste

1 medium head red cabbage (about 1½ pounds), cored and thinly sliced

1 cup fresh cranberries, coarsely chopped, or ½ cup whole dried sweetened cranberries

1 large ripe but firm pear, such as Anjou, unpeeled and cut into matchsticks

Before You Start If you like the tart crunch of raw cranberries, they really add an unexpected twist to this slaw, but if they're too tart for you, dried sweetened cranberries work very well.

1. In a large bowl, whisk together the shallot, maple syrup, cider vinegar, yogurt, and salt.

2. Toss the cabbage, cranberries, and pear into the bowl with the dressing. Adjust seasoning to taste and let sit for at least 30 minutes and up to several hours to allow flavors to blend before serving.

Variation See Seven More Things to Do with Maple (page 52) for another way to use this dressing.

Tending the Sugarbush

David Marvin, sugarmaker,
Butternut Mountain Farm

"Stewardship is a far greater aspiration than ownership."

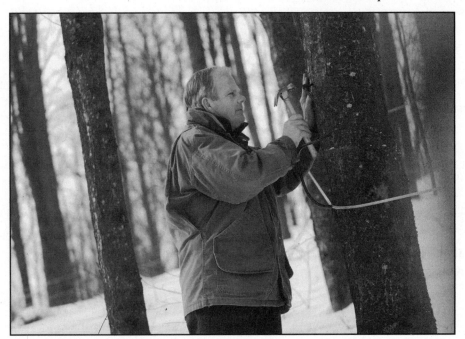

*t*o those who would grumble about Vermont's "fifth season"—the early spring weeks during which dirt roads meet snowmelt and hubcaps are swallowed whole by the mud—sugarmaker David Marvin says simply, "Mud season is why we have maple."

Even the most crotchety Vermonter probably wouldn't trade maple for mud season, when the first sap plinks into buckets hung from the maple trunks or starts coursing through the blue veins of a sugarbush pipeline system. That's when the call goes out, "The sap's running, the sap's running! Get down to the sugarhouse and help boil."

Mud season is a long way off on a freezing winter day when David ventures into the sugarbush to check on his trees. Butternut Mountain is quiet with snow, a few flakes swirling down here and there as branches shiver. Late winter is when you check the lines, trim the deadwood, and "make sure the young trees that show promise have room to grow," David explains. He points to a healthy maple with "a nice big crown, full all the way around with lots of live branches and twigs." In contrast, a fork is a sign of weakness, he says, looking up at another tree that splits high above his head. "I should cut it, but it's so hard to a cut a maple," he shakes his head. "I hate to do it."

David has known these trees for most of his life. Like three quarters of Vermont, the land around Butternut Mountain in Johnson had been cleared by settlers, and when he was young it was pasture transitioning back to forest. "I can remember picking blackberries up here and being scared of bears," he says. "These were all young trees when I was a kid." Except for one tree, a huge, craggy maple. "I figure it's been around since the Civil War," he says, laying a hand on the bark. "I like this tree a lot. I've been tapping it for thirty-five years. It's a pretty unusual tree."

The trees are part of the Marvin family's Butternut Mountain Farm, which includes some twelve thousand taps over three hundred acres. The syrup was the start of the family's successful business, but the company has grown far beyond it to become not just the largest handler of Vermont syrup but also a major processor and distributor of maple products nationwide under its own brand and a number of national names, including Shelburne Farms.

The family has maple syrup in its blood. David's father was a renowned maple researcher and chair of the botany department at the University of Vermont, where David earned a degree in forestry. "My goal my whole life was to make a living from maple," he says. "From the perspective of working the landscape, sugaring is wonderful because it doesn't diminish the resource . . . and it's a wondrous flavor that hasn't changed since the Native Americans showed us how to do it."

We might do well to take other lessons from the Native Americans, David believes, to appreciate that we are "only part of an intricate web of life, death, evolution, growth, and struggle that is yet to be truly understood." His first grandchild will be introduced this year to the sweet scent of the sugarhouse. He hopes that when she is grown the trees will still be there for her to care for and that she, too, will see, as he puts it, "that stewardship is a far greater aspiration than ownership."

Maple-Braised Red Cabbage with Pear and Cranberries

Now for the warm version. Both the slaw and the braise go well with our Maple and Black Pepper Chicken (page 48) and make a colorful side for a holiday roast turkey or ham. ◇ *Serves: 6*

1 tablespoon olive oil

3 medium shallots, thinly sliced

1 medium head red cabbage (about 1½ pounds), cored and cut into rough 1-inch-square chunks

2 teaspoons coarse kosher salt plus more to taste

¼ cup pure maple syrup

¼ cup apple cider or natural apple juice

3 tablespoons cider vinegar

1 cup whole fresh cranberries, coarsely chopped, or ½ cup whole dried sweetened cranberries

1 large ripe but firm pear, such as Anjou, unpeeled and cut into matchsticks

Before You Start   At the Inn, Rick likes to smoke maple syrup in a Weber over wood chips for hours so that it absorbs a lightly smoky scent and flavor, heightening the sugarhouse aroma some people already taste in maple syrup. If you want to, add a dash of a bottled smoke product, such as Liquid Smoke, to this braise at the end for a similar effect.

1. Heat a large sauté pan or skillet over medium heat and add the olive oil. When the olive oil is hot, add the shallots and cook, stirring occasionally, until golden, about 3–4 minutes.

2. Add the cabbage and salt to the pan and cook, stirring occasionally, until the cabbage is wilted, about 5–6 minutes. Add the maple syrup, apple cider, and cider vinegar to the pan and bring to a simmer. Simmer uncovered for 20 minutes.

3. Add the cranberries and pear. Cover the pan and simmer for another 15–20 minutes until the cabbage is completely soft. Adjust seasoning to taste and serve.

Maple-Chipotle Scallops

A little heat from the south meets the cool sweetness of the north to give nice, fat sea scallops a smoky-sweet touch. We serve these over rice or noodles with crisp, lightly steamed broccoli or green beans. ◇ **Serves: 4**

½ cup freshly squeezed orange juice

1 tablespoon freshly squeezed lime juice

¼ cup pure maple syrup

½ chipotle chili pepper in adobo sauce, finely minced, or more to taste

1 teaspoon adobo sauce or more to taste

2 teaspoons coarse kosher salt plus more to taste

1 tablespoon olive oil

1½ pounds large sea scallops (about 4–5 per person), patted dry

Before You Start   Small cans of chipotle chili peppers in adobo sauce can be found in the Mexican section of many supermarkets, and they keep forever in the refrigerator (see Venison Chili, page 152, for another use). Make sure that your scallops are "dry," which means they have not been soaked in a solution that encourages them to retain water and makes it very hard to get a nice, seared crust. We also strongly recommend fresh scallops, not frozen or previously frozen ones, which never brown as well as fresh.

1. In a small bowl, whisk together the orange juice, lime juice, maple syrup, minced chili pepper, adobo sauce, and 1 teaspoon of the salt. Set aside.

2. In a large sauté pan or skillet set over medium-high heat, heat the olive oil until almost smoking. Make sure the scallops are very dry, and season them on both sides with the remaining teaspoon of salt.

3. Place the scallops flat side down in the pan (they should sizzle), and cook them for about 2–3 minutes without moving them until a nice golden brown crust develops. Turn them over and cook them the same way on the other side until they are just cooked through. Remove them to a plate.

4. Take the pan off the heat and pour in the sauce. Put the pan back over medium heat and simmer for 4–5 minutes to reduce the sauce. Return the scallops to the pan and toss to coat them in the sauce and heat them through, 1–2 minutes. Adjust seasoning to taste and serve immediately.

Maple and
Black Pepper Chicken

[photograph 4]

The sweetness of maple is balanced nicely by the cider vinegar and the light heat of black pepper in the sauce for this golden-skinned chicken. Enjoy it for a weeknight supper with crusty bread and a green salad dressed with our Cider Vinaigrette (page 218) or the Red Cabbage, Pear, and Cranberry Slaw (page 43), or try it with Maple-Roasted Butternut Squash Puree or Soup (page 202). ◇**Serves: 4**

1½ teaspoons whole black peppercorns

1 chicken, about 4–4½-pounds, cut into six pieces: two legs, two thighs, two bone-in breast halves with wings

2 teaspoons coarse kosher salt plus more to taste

1 tablespoon olive oil

1 large shallot, finely chopped

2 tablespoons finely chopped fresh thyme leaves

⅓ cup cider vinegar

½ cup pure maple syrup

1. Preheat the oven to 375°F with a rack set in the second-highest position. With a mortar and pestle or a spice grinder, coarsely grind the peppercorns and set them aside.

2. Pat the chicken pieces dry and season them well with 1½ teaspoons of the salt. In a large, heavy-bottomed sauté pan or skillet set over medium-high heat, heat the olive oil for 3–4 minutes until shimmering. Put the chicken breasts into the pan skin side down and cook for about 7–9 minutes, without moving, until the skin is golden brown. Remove the chicken to a baking dish or roasting pan large enough to hold all the pieces. Next, brown the thighs and drumsticks, turning so the skin is evenly browned, up to 10 minutes.

3. Add the thighs and drumsticks to the baking dish and put the chicken in the oven. (Reserve the pan.) Roast for about 30–35 minutes until the chicken flesh closest to the bone is opaque. An instant-read thermometer should register about 165°F for the breasts and 175°F for the thighs and legs.

4. While the chicken is roasting, make the sauce in the reserved pan. Discard all but 2 tablespoons of the fat and set the pan over medium-high heat. Add the shallot, thyme, and the remaining ½ teaspoon of salt, and cook, stirring, for 1–2 minutes or just until the shallot starts to color. Add the vinegar and simmer for 1–2 minutes, using a spatula to scrape any brown bits from the bottom of the pan. Add the maple syrup and ground peppercorns and simmer for about 8–10 minutes until the sauce is reduced by about half. Adjust seasoning to taste. Spoon the sauce over the chicken and serve immediately.

Calf's Liver with Sage, Shallots, and Maple-Vinegar Sauce

*Although home cooks today shy away from cooking liver because of squeamishness and fear of fat, calf's liver packs a huge nutritional bang for the buck (there was a reason mothers used to encourage their children to eat liver), and, prepared well, it is also delicious. We like to cook with it, and other less common cuts, because we believe that fully utilizing an animal is the best way to honor the food it has provided us. This savory-sweet liver is especially good served over mashed potatoes. ◇ **Serves: 4***

¼ cup all-purpose flour

1 teaspoon coarse kosher salt plus more to taste

Freshly ground black pepper to taste

1 pound calf's liver, cut into slices about ½ inch thick, or 1 pound chicken livers, trimmed of any membranes

1–2 tablespoons olive oil

3 tablespoons unsalted butter

4 small shallots, trimmed with root end left intact so that they can be cut into thirds and hold together

12 fresh sage leaves

2 tablespoons cider vinegar

½ cup chicken stock, preferably low sodium

2 tablespoons pure maple syrup

Before You Start   Calf's liver is the most delicate and smooth-textured of all livers you can buy, but chicken livers also work nicely with this sauce. Either way, make sure not to overcook them or you will be eating rubber.

1. Pour the flour into a shallow rimmed plate or pie pan and whisk in the salt and a few grinds of pepper. Pat the liver dry and dredge it lightly in the flour mixture.

2. Heat a large sauté pan or skillet over medium-high heat. Add 1 tablespoon of olive oil to lightly coat the bottom of the pan. When the olive oil is hot, cook the liver, in batches if necessary to avoid crowding the pan, 1–2 minutes per side just until deep golden brown. Set the liver aside on a plate and cover it with foil to keep it warm.

3. Melt the butter in the pan until foamy. Add the shallots to the pan and cook, stirring occasionally, for 3–4 minutes until the shallots are softened. Add the sage and cook for another 2–3 minutes until the shallot is golden and the sage is crisp. Add the vinegar and deglaze the pan, stirring to scrape up any brown bits.

4. Add the chicken stock and maple syrup to the pan and bring to a simmer. Simmer for 2–3 minutes to reduce the sauce a little. Adjust seasoning to taste and return the liver to the pan to warm it through and coat it with the sauce. Serve immediately.

Seven More Things to Do with Maple

Here are some of our favorite quick ways to add the special flavor of maple to our food. Grade B is fine in any of these.

- For Warm Maple and Tart Cherry Brie, split a small wheel of Brie through the middle horizontally. On the bottom half, sprinkle about 2 tablespoons of chopped dried sweetened tart cherries or cranberries and then drizzle with 2 tablespoons of maple syrup. Top with the remaining half of the Brie, wrap in foil, and bake for 10 minutes at 300°F until just soft and warm. Serve with bread or crackers.

- Brush bacon with maple syrup and broil for Maple-Glazed Bacon.

- For Maple-Ginger Roasted Root Vegetables, cut 2 pounds of assorted peeled root vegetables (beets, parsnips, carrots, turnips, or rutabagas) into 1-inch cubes and toss them with ¼ cup each of maple syrup and olive oil and about 2 tablespoons of fresh, peeled ginger cut into matchsticks. Add salt to taste and roast at 425°F until tender, about 40 minutes.

- Swirl together equal parts maple syrup and mustard for a Maple-Mustard Glaze for salmon, pork, or ham. Add a touch of horseradish for a bigger kick.

- Use the sauce from Maple-Chipotle Scallops (page 47) to coat sweet potato wedges for Maple-Chipotle Sweet Potato Oven Fries, roasted at 400°F until soft, about 25–30 minutes.

- Whisk up a quick Maple Barbecue Sauce with ½ cup of medium-bodied ale, ½ cup of maple syrup, ¼ cup of cider vinegar, ½ cup of ketchup, 1 teaspoon of paprika, and 1 teaspoon of coarse kosher salt, and simmer for 10 minutes. Broil or grill chicken, pork, beef, or salmon and brush the sauce on for the last 5 minutes of cooking.

- Toss crisp, steamed green beans (or broccoli florets) with some crumbled bacon, slivered toasted almonds, and Maple-Yogurt Dressing (page 43) to make Creamy Maple and Bacon Green Beans.

Early
Spring
and
Summer
Greens

- Springtime Eggs Benedict with Wild Greens and Mushrooms
- Inn at Shelburne Farms Pickled Ramps
- Market-Garden Baby Vegetables with Spring Herb Mayonnaise
- Cream of Spring Soup
- Wilted Dandelion Greens with Bacon and Croutons
- The Whole-Pea Salad with Deviled Farm Barn Eggs
- Fiddlehead and Fresh Herb Tart
- Pasta with Sweet Peas and Morels
- A Vermont Spring Tonic: Rhubarb-Citrus Soda
- Rhubarb and Yogurt Fool

*a*fter a long, dark, cold winter, Vermonters are greeted by the slosh of mud season and then a mere snippet of spring. Dirt roads turn into quagmires, but it's better to walk anyway so that you can appreciate the newborn green brushing the tips of the trees. The translucent emerald shimmer that rises over the Vermont landscape in early April is one of the first signs that warmer weather is finally on the way. But for those who lived off the land for centuries before us, the receding ice and snow had already revealed early spring treasures: watercress trailing in chilly streams, plant roots full of stored winter energy, cattail shoots, and tender tree buds.

Like the native Abenaki, when spring finally arrives, we crave all that is green and growing: the delicate curl of the fiddlehead fern; the fragrant, slender wild leeks known as ramps; the reliable rebirth of garden perennials like rhubarb, lemony sorrel, and asparagus. The original Shelburne Farms greenhouses fed those needs by producing early-season vegetables including asparagus and peas in a state-of-the-art complex that included twenty-five thousand square feet of interconnected steam-heated units built from glass and iron on brick foundations—although during World War I the Webbs curtailed production as part of the war effort.

As May warms into June and the sun moves slowly higher in the sky, fiddleheads and the first soft dandelion leaves make way

for tangy wood sorrel and the succulent crunch of purslane.
In gardens, dark pink rhubarb stalks poke their heads up under a
curve of green leaf and the earliest peas start climbing toward
the light as tender lettuces and baby greens sprout bravely into a
fresh, new world.

A Note on Wild Greens

As with any wild edibles, take great care to eat only plants that you can conclusively identify and that do not grow where they may have been sprayed with chemicals. It is also critical to know enough about a particular plant to understand how to harvest so that you do not adversely affect the population of that plant. Shelburne Farms field naturalist Matt Kolan recommends *Identifying and Harvesting Edible and Medicinal Plants in Wild (and Not So Wild) Places* by Steve Brill as a good place to start learning.

Springtime Eggs Benedict with Wild Greens and Mushrooms

[photograph 5]

David Hugo was head chef at Shelburne Farms for five years, but he started out as the breakfast chef creating this kind of seasonal, locally inspired dish. David forages his own ingredients and, ideally, he says, this recipe would use pheasant backs, an early-season mushroom often found near beds of wild leeks, or ramps. He would serve the eggs over O-Bread Bakery's brioche. ◇ **Serves: 4**

8 ounces fiddlehead ferns (see Tip, page 58) or 1 pound asparagus, tough ends trimmed, cut into 1-inch lengths

1 tablespoon olive oil

16 small ramps, dark green tops trimmed, bulbs cut in half lengthwise, or ½ cup chives, cut into 1-inch lengths

8 ounces pheasant back or cremini mushrooms, thinly sliced

½ teaspoon coarse kosher salt plus more to taste

1½ cups heavy cream

4 ounces (about 1 cup) grated cheddar (see Before You Start)

Freshly ground black pepper to taste

1 tablespoon freshly squeezed lemon juice

8 large eggs (see Tip, page 58)

4 soft rolls or buns, split and lightly toasted if desired

Before You Start Even without fiddleheads, ramps, and pheasant backs, you can still make a wonderful version of this Benedict with cremini (brown button) mushrooms, asparagus, and chives; the last two are both harbingers of the growing season in their own right. For the sauce, use fairly young but sharp cheddar, such as Shelburne Farms six- or nine-month. This is a recipe best made with help, as there are a few things going on at the same time. This recipe calls for lightly cooked eggs—please see Some General Guidelines to Our Recipes page xv, for further information.

1. Put a medium pot of salted water fitted with a steamer insert on to boil. Steam the fiddleheads for 5 minutes just until tender. (Asparagus may need a minute or two more.) Set the fiddleheads aside, but leave the pot of water on the burner on low heat.

2. In a medium sauté pan or skillet set over medium-high heat, heat the olive oil until hot. Add the ramps and cook, stirring occasionally, for 2–3 minutes until they start to soften. (If you are using chives, hold those until step 5.) Add the mushrooms and the salt and cook, stirring occasionally, until the mushrooms have given up their liquid and turned golden, and they make a squeaking noise against the pan, 5–6 minutes. Toss in the reserved fiddleheads, adjust seasoning to taste, and cover the pan to keep the vegetables warm.

3. While the vegetables are cooking, bring the heavy cream to a gentle simmer in a medium saucepan and simmer for about 12–15 minutes to reduce by about one third. Take the pan off the heat and stir in the cheddar until the sauce is smooth. Adjust seasoning to taste and cover to keep warm.

4. Increase the heat under the pot of water and add the lemon juice to the pot. When the water is simmering, crack one of the eggs into a large slotted spoon set over a small bowl to strain off any thin strands of white, and then gently lower the egg into the simmering water. Repeat with a second egg immediately. Cook the eggs for about 3 minutes for a medium-soft yolk. Repeat with the remaining eggs.

5. Serve each pair of poached eggs as soon as they are cooked. Place each egg on a roll half, top with a spoonful of the vegetables and, if using chives, sprinkle those on now. Top each with a small ladleful of cheddar sauce and serve.

Tip: *When selecting fiddleheads, be sure they are the new growing tips of the ostrich fern (Matteuccia struthiopteris, also known as Matteuccia pensylvanica). The new growth of a few other ferns is edible but is not as tasty and may cause stomach upset. Unfurled ferns should not be eaten at all. Look for a tight coil about an inch in diameter with an inch or two of stem beyond the coil. Rub off any brown, papery chaff before cooking, and wash the fiddleheads well in several changes of cold water.*

Tip: *The freshest eggs will yield the neatest poached eggs because their whites are thickest.*

Prepare-Ahead Tip: *A restaurant trick is to pre-poach the eggs, hold them in a bowl of cold water, and then pop them back in simmering water for 20–30 seconds to warm right before serving.*

Inn at Shelburne Farms Pickled Ramps

[photograph 3]

When the first wild leeks poke up through the mud in April, Vermonters take to the hills to gently dig up the white bulbs with their pink-purple stalks and dark green leaves. Ramps, as they are commonly called, can be used anywhere a scallion might be, but they offer a softer bite. Rick created this tangy-sweet pickle to keep them around after their season has passed. He serves them with his charcuterie board, to garnish roast chicken, and in a salad with roasted beets and goat cheese. They add a wonderfully unexpected touch to a cheese plate and are a great Vermont substitute for the classic pickled onion in our Green Mountain Ploughman's Lunch (page 21). They also go especially well with Sausage Rolls (page 169). ◇ ***Makes: 1 pint (can be easily doubled)***

20 small ramps (about 10 ounces), trimmed to 1 inch of greens and cleaned well, or about 10 medium shallots, peeled, with root end trimmed but left intact

1 cup cider vinegar

¼ cup honey

¼ cup sugar

1 scant teaspoon finely minced dried chile de arbol or crushed red pepper

1 teaspoon whole black peppercorns

1 teaspoon whole fennel seeds

1 teaspoon whole coriander seeds

1 bay leaf

Before You Start Although you could substitute scallions here, we prefer using shallots if ramps are not available. You may want to cut the shallots in half when you serve them. Chiles de arbol are smoky, fairly hot peppers that can be bought dried at some specialty stores. (See Sources, page 273). We do these as refrigerator pickles, so no need to boil the jar after it is filled, but do make sure it is very clean before filling and use a tight-fitting lid.

1. Prepare a large bowl of ice water. Bring a medium pot of salted water to a boil over high heat, add the ramps, and boil for 2 minutes (3 minutes for shallots). Drain immediately and plunge the ramps into the ice water to stop cooking.

2. In the same medium pot (emptied of water), bring the cider vinegar, honey, sugar, chile de arbol, peppercorns, fennel, coriander, and bay leaf to a simmer, and then remove the pot from the heat.

3. Put the drained ramps into a clean pint jar. Pour the hot pickling liquid into the jar. When the mixture is cool, cover it tightly and refrigerate for at least 12 hours before eating. The pickles can be stored in the refrigerator for about a month.

Putting Down Roots

Matt Kolan, naturalist, Shelburne Farms

"Foraging is one way of getting back into natural cycles; sometimes it's just about celebration of the landscape so that you can feel like you're a part of it."

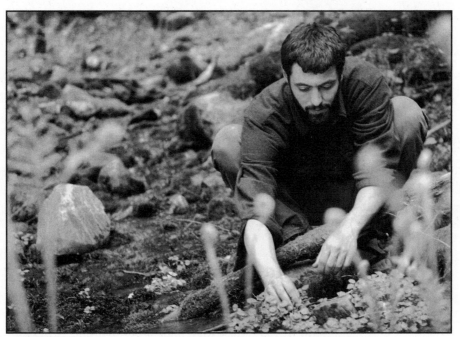

*i*n the middle of a muddy pathway, Shelburne Farms field naturalist Matt Kolan crouches down to point out a tiny green nub pushing up into the pale sunshine. It is the very end of March and the spot of green is the first sign of this year's fiddleheads, the tender tops of the ostrich fern, which are probably valued as much for being one of the earliest edible greens as for their pleasantly mild but unremarkable flavor.

In a few short weeks, the swelling sprout will have continued its path upward and crowned the top of a fuzzy green-brown stalk with a beautifully curled tip, reminiscent of the scroll at the top of a fiddle's neck. The window for fiddleheads is short; once they unfurl, they should not be eaten. They represent the brief moment when the light softens under a bright-blue, winter-crisp sky while the fields remain bordered with snow where trees cast cool shadows along their edges.

Wild edibles are just beginning to reemerge and it takes a keen eye and an open mind to see the life ready to spring from the landscape. Walking on through a nippy breeze, boots squelching through the mud, Matt explains that roots can be dug from the thawing earth or out of chilly wetland marshes: those of Jerusalem artichokes to be eaten as tubers, of burdock to be brewed into spring tonics, or of cattails to be pounded into a kind of flour. Other plants—like watercress—are just starting to grow in streams swollen with melting snow and soon cattails will produce shoots that taste like cucumber when eaten raw.

He kneels to investigate some fresh leaves, a circle of deep green against the browns of mud and dry leaves. The tiny leaves in the center are the first new growth of a variety of dock, perhaps curly or bitter dock. He looks at the spent stalks nearby to see if he can recognize the seed pods and determine if the leaves are edible, but is not quite sure. "Being out in the woods always offers new lessons and patterns," Matt says, "and I'm always humbled by how much there is to learn, how intricate the connections are, and how little I really know."

Matt is a graduate of the field naturalist program at the University of Vermont where he now teaches and is researching his doctorate. For the last few years, he has also worked with Shelburne Farms leading field walks, helping with land management, and running educational programs like a weekend of traditional skills during which participants craft their own tools, learn to track animals, and gather wild edibles for a largely foraged meal.

He hopes to "get the community engaged in the land through connecting them with its natural cycles and rhythms," he explains. "Foraging is one way of getting back into natural cycles," he continues, but "sometimes it's just about celebration of the landscape so that you can feel like you're a part of it. Really getting to know a place so you know when and where to go see things like the migration of the salamander from the forested uplands to the wetlands where they breed. Or where to see the spring ephemerals—the wildflowers like trillium, trout lily, and hepatica—that bloom only briefly in late April and early May."

Matt urges his students to make a daily practice of observing one place in nature. Pick a spot: a corner of woods or even your backyard. Devote a little time every day to sitting and watching it "in the rain, in the sun, in the morning, and the evening—to see how a place adapts to the changing season," he suggests. "I think there are a lot of lessons we can learn about how we live our daily lives, like the gracefulness with which species other than humans make transitions between seasons," he says.

Some recently returned Canada geese call to each other in a nearby field. Looking up, Matt spies a robin wrestling with a dark-red fuzzy cone of staghorn sumac berries. "Robins can often be seen eating sumac in the early spring when there's not much else around," he says, and explains that he likes to steep the berries in maple sap collected from trees around his house. The resulting citrusy, lightly sweet tea is a taste of Vermont at a very specific time of year, and it carries with it the distinctive and delicious flavor of what Matt calls "the beauty of rooting yourself in a place."

Market-Garden Baby Vegetables with Spring Herb Mayonnaise

*This is not so much a recipe as an inspiration to go to your local farmers'
market at the dawn of a new season and fill your basket with the most tender,
newborn baby vegetables you can find: creamy baby turnips, chubby watermelon
radishes, miniature yellow and orange carrots with feathery topknots, luminously
green peas with their flowering tendrils, and tiny marble-size new potatoes. Buy
some fresh farm eggs and herbs too, for the mayonnaise.*

*We hope that you will feel as Rick did when he first began working at
Shelburne Farms and the Market-Garden vegetable salad became—to his surprise—
his favorite dish on the menu. It was simply a plate of perfect, crisp, just-picked
vegetables dressed with a fresh herb mayonnaise; showered with delicate tarragon,
chervil, mint, basil, and cilantro leaves; and finished with a dash of champagne
vinegar and a crunch of Maldon sea salt. "It's just crazy that a plate of raw
vegetables could be so good," he says, shaking his head in awe.* ◇ ***Makes: 1½ cups***

2 large egg yolks

1½ teaspoons Dijon mustard

½ teaspoon coarse kosher salt

2 teaspoons freshly squeezed
lemon juice

2 teaspoons white wine vinegar or
champagne vinegar

1 cup light-tasting oil such as
grapeseed or a light olive

1 finely minced teaspoon each of
3–4 herbs such as tarragon, chervil,
mint, basil, or cilantro

Assorted small, raw spring
vegetables (see Before You Start)

Before You Start You can use any small, raw spring
vegetables, but try to find a variety of shape, color, and texture.
Trim them lightly (no peeling necessary), leaving a little green
on root vegetables like radishes and carrots. The only vegetables
that Rick cooks are the tiny new potatoes, which he steams
briefly. This recipe calls for uncooked eggs—please see Some
General Guidelines to Our Recipes, page xv, for further
information.

1. Put the egg yolks, mustard, salt, lemon juice, and vinegar in a
blender and blend until smooth and creamy.

2. With the blender running, gradually drizzle the oil through the
hole in the blender lid until the mayonnaise is thick and creamy.

3. Scrape the mayonnaise into a small bowl and stir in the herbs.
Adjust seasoning to taste and serve with the vegetables. The mayonnaise
can be kept in the refrigerator for a day or two.

Cream of Spring Soup

We borrowed this alluring recipe name (but not the recipe that goes with it) from a Vermont classic, Mrs. Appleyard, the pen name of Louise Andrews Kent, who wrote a series of endearingly quirky cooking columns that were originally published in Vermont Life *magazine and then in book form in the early 1960s. This soup is the most amazing vibrant green. It is similar to a spring pea soup served at the Inn with shreds of sweet crab, brioche croutons, and a drizzle of brown butter—a fine way to dress it up for company if you choose.* ◇ *Makes: 4 cups*

1 tablespoon unsalted butter

4 small shallots, minced

4 cups water

1½ teaspoons coarse kosher salt plus more to taste

4 cups fresh shelled peas or 1 (16-ounce) bag frozen peas

15–20 sorrel leaves (about 2 ounces), tough stems removed

20 butter lettuce leaves

1 cup whole milk

1–2 teaspoons freshly squeezed lemon juice plus more to taste

Before You Start If you're using fresh peas, the smallest, most tender, early-season ones will work best. The peas add body to the soup, but their starch also adds a slight grittiness, which is why we recommend pushing the soup through a sieve. It's a bit of a chore but worth it for the beautifully smooth texture. The soup can be served warm or chilled.

1. In a 3-quart saucepan set over medium heat, melt the butter until foamy and then add the shallots. Cook, stirring occasionally, until the shallots are soft, 3–5 minutes.

2. Add the water and salt to the pot and increase the heat to high. Bring the pot to a boil and add the peas. Cook until the peas are tender, about 5–7 minutes.

3. Strain the peas and shallots through a fine-meshed sieve, reserving the cooking liquid. Put half the peas and shallots into a blender and set the other half aside in a bowl. Add half the sorrel, half the lettuce, ½ cup of the milk, and ½ cup of the cooking liquid, and blend until smooth. (Take care when blending hot liquids—see the Tip on page 14.) Pour the blended soup back through the sieve into the saucepan, pressing with a spatula to get as much liquid through as possible.

4. Blend the remaining peas, shallots, sorrel, lettuce, and milk and strain the mixture through the sieve back into the pot.

5. Rewarm the soup gently and add the lemon juice, starting with 1 teaspoon. Adjust seasoning to taste and add more lemon juice as desired.

Prepare-Ahead Tip: You can make the soup up to a couple of days ahead through step 4. When ready to serve, start at step 5, skipping the warming step if you're serving the soup chilled.

Wilted Dandelion Greens with Bacon and Croutons

Dandelion greens must be gathered at the beginning of the season, before they bloom, when they're still tender and only mildly astringent. The cultivated variety are also best picked young, although that does not always seem to be the case with bunches found in stores. If the leaves are on the large side, be prepared for a tannic bite, which has its own charm but is not for everyone. This makes a nice lunch or light supper with a bowl of creamy soup like Tomato-Cheddar Soup (page 15), Maple-Roasted Butternut Squash Puree or Soup (page 202), or Celery Root Soup with Blue Cheese (page 190). ◇ **Serves: 4 as a side dish or warm salad**

5–6 slices (about 6 ounces) thick-cut bacon, diced

Olive oil as needed

2 thick slices hearty, country-style bread, trimmed of hard crusts and cut into ½-inch cubes (about 1–1½ cups)

¼ teaspoon coarse kosher salt plus more to taste

2 medium shallots, thinly sliced

2 tablespoons cider vinegar

1½ pounds dandelion greens, cleaned, trimmed of any tough stems, and cut into 1-inch ribbons (see Tip, page 67)

Freshly ground black pepper to taste

Before You Start   Small leaves of chicory or frisée will substitute for dandelion greens.

1. In a large sauté pan or skillet, fry the bacon until crisp. Remove the bacon to a plate lined with paper towel. Pour off and reserve any bacon fat in excess of 3 tablespoons. (If you have less than 3 tablespoons, add olive oil to the pan.)

2. Put the pan with the bacon fat back over medium heat and add the bread to the pan with the salt. Cook, turning occasionally, until the croutons are golden on all sides, about 5–6 minutes. Remove them to a plate.

3. Put a tablespoon of reserved bacon fat if you have it—or olive oil if you don't—back into the pan and set it over medium heat. Add the shallots and cook until golden, 2–3 minutes. Add the cider vinegar to the pan and simmer for 30 seconds.

4. With tongs, add the dandelion greens to the pan and toss a few times to evenly wilt them. Taste to make sure they are tender enough for you, since this will vary greatly depending on the age of the greens. If they are still tough or very bitter, add a little water, lower the heat, cover, and allow them to cook for about 5 minutes. Adjust seasoning to taste.

5. Remove the greens from the pan and divide evenly among four plates. Top with the bacon and croutons. Serve immediately.

> **Tip:** To cut large greens into ribbons, lay a few on top of each other and roll them tightly lengthwise. Now slice across the roll.

The Whole-Pea Salad with Deviled Farm Barn Eggs

[photograph 6]

When the first pea shoots make their way up through still-chilly soil, it is worth a celebration—or at least a salad created in their honor. Since eggs are also a symbol of spring and new life and, as the days lengthen, the hens in the Children's Farmyard at Shelburne Farms lay faster and eggs are plentiful, it seemed natural to pair the two. Besides, I have never met anyone who doesn't love a deviled egg. ◇ ***Serves: 4***

For the deviled eggs and salad

1 teaspoon whole mustard seeds

4 large hard-cooked eggs (see Tip, page 69)

½ teaspoon Dijon mustard

2 teaspoons mayonnaise

½ teaspoon freshly squeezed lemon juice

¼ teaspoon coarse kosher salt plus more to taste

Freshly ground black pepper to taste

1 tablespoon olive oil

¼ pound tender pea greens and flowers if possible (see Before You Start)

¼ pound (about ¾ cup) fresh shelled peas, blanched (see Tip, page 69), or frozen peas, thawed

8 small radishes, trimmed and halved

For the dressing

1 tablespoon freshly squeezed lemon juice

¾ teaspoon Dijon mustard

3 tablespoons extra-virgin olive oil

8 large leaves fresh basil

Before You Start Early-season pea greens—sometimes called shoots or sprouts—with flowers and tendrils are beautiful and usually tender, but they can also be woody and tough. You can break the more tender branches from the tougher stems if necessary, but buy extra if you think you may need to do that. If you can't find pea greens, any of the larger fresh sprouts, like sunflower, will work nicely in this salad; they will not need to be cooked.

1. Make the deviled eggs: In a small skillet set over medium-high heat, toast the mustard seeds until fragrant, about 3 minutes. Remove them to a mortar and pestle or spice grinder and crush them coarsely. Set aside.

2. Peel the eggs and slice them in half lengthwise. Scoop out the yolks into a small bowl. Add the Dijon mustard, mayonnaise, lemon juice, ⅛ teaspoon of the salt, a few grinds of pepper, and ½ teaspoon of the crushed mustard seed, and mix well. Taste and add more salt and mustard seed as desired. Fill the egg whites back up with the yolk mixture and set aside.

3. Make the pea greens: In a medium skillet or sauté pan set over medium heat, heat the olive oil until hot. Add the pea greens to the pan. Sprinkle with the remaining ⅛ teaspoon of salt. Cook the greens, stirring, until just wilted, 2–3 minutes.

4. *Make the dressing:* In a small bowl, whisk together the lemon juice and mustard. Gradually drizzle in the olive oil while whisking until the dressing is emulsified. Thinly slice the basil leaves and stir them into the dressing. (Don't slice the leaves ahead of time, as sliced basil leaves darken quickly.)

5. *Finish the salad:* Divide the pea greens among four plates. Scatter with the peas, halved radishes, and a tablespoon of dressing per plate. Set two deviled egg halves on each plate and serve.

Tip: To make pretty hard-cooked eggs, you actually want to use older eggs, which peel much more easily than fresh. The other key, as many food science experts have pointed out, is not to let the eggs actually boil, which is too extreme a cooking temperature and may cause that ugly gray-green ring around the yolk. Put the eggs in a roomy pot and add just enough cold water to cover them. Add a generous pinch of salt. Bring the pot just to a boil and take it off the heat. Cover the pot and let it sit for 6–7 minutes. Remove the eggs to an ice-water bath, let them cool for 5 minutes, and then remove them from the water. These eggs should still have a slightly soft yolk. If you prefer a harder-cooked yolk, let the eggs sit in the hot water for another 3–4 minutes.

Tip: To blanch fresh peas, bring a large pot of salted water to a boil, add the peas, and cook for 1–2 minutes until just tender. Drain the peas and then shock them in a big bowl of ice water to stop the cooking.

Prepare-Ahead Tip: The deviled eggs can be made up to a day ahead and kept in the refrigerator.

Fiddlehead and Fresh Herb Tart

The green and yellow tones and sprightly flavors of this tart are a sign of spring all by themselves. The tart really shows off the fanciful curl of the fiddlehead, but it is also lovely with the tips and tender stems of asparagus, one of the first cultivated harvests of the season in Vermont. ◇ ***Serves: 12 as an appetizer, 4–6 as a light main dish***

1 (10 by 10-inch) sheet frozen puff pastry (half of a 17.3-ounce box)

6 ounces (about 1 cup) fiddleheads (see Tip, page 58) or asparagus tips and ½-inch pieces of tender stalks

2 tablespoons water

2 tablespoons minced, assorted fresh herbs, such as flat-leaf parsley, marjoram, basil, tarragon, or chervil

2 garlic cloves, finely minced

1½ teaspoons finely grated lemon zest

3–4 ounces crumbled (about 1 cup) soft, fresh goat cheese

1 tablespoon extra-virgin olive oil

½ teaspoon coarse kosher salt

1 large egg yolk whisked with 1 teaspoon water

Before You Start   If you don't have a microwave, steam the fiddleheads according to step 1 of the Springtime Eggs Benedict recipe (page 57). If you have any finely ground sea salt, such as Maldon, around, this is a wonderful place to use it.

1. Thaw the puff pastry according to package directions. Preheat the oven to 375°F with a rack set in the lower third of the oven. Lightly grease a cookie sheet.

2. Put the fiddleheads in a small bowl with 2 tablespoons of water. Cover with plastic wrap with a hole poked in it. Microwave on high for 2 minutes or until the fiddleheads are just barely tender. (They will cook more in the oven.) Drain and pat the fiddleheads dry.

3. Unfold the thawed puff pastry sheet on the prepared cookie sheet and roll it gently into a 14 by 10-inch rectangle. With a sharp knife, make a ½-inch diagonal cut in from each corner of the puff pastry sheet. Lightly brush the edges of the rectangle with water and fold in half-inch borders on each side to form an edge for the tart. Prick the bottom of the tart with a fork about a dozen times.

4. Sprinkle the bottom of the tart evenly with the minced herbs, garlic, and lemon zest. Spread the fiddleheads evenly over the tart, followed by the goat cheese. Drizzle the olive oil over the top and then sprinkle the salt evenly over the filling.

5. Brush the tart border with the egg yolk and water mixture. Bake for about 15 minutes or until the pastry is golden. Cool on a rack for 5 minutes before cutting into pieces and serving warm or at room temperature.

Pasta with Sweet Peas and Morels

This dish fairly sings of spring with the sweet peas and tarragon balanced by rich, woodsy morels and a light cream sauce. Fresh morels are among the first and most highly prized mushrooms found in Vermont every year; their distinctive honeycombed caps pop up from May through September in woods and even old apple orchards. After we developed this recipe for the cookbook, Rick started serving it at the Inn. He enriches it with a dollop of crème fraîche and uses finely minced preserved lemon rather than lemon zest. ◇ **Serves: 4–6**

10 small fresh morels, halved lengthwise, or ½ ounce dried morels (see page 109 for cleaning tip)

1 tablespoon olive oil

2 medium shallots, thinly sliced

¾ cup dry white wine

1½ cups heavy cream

½ pound (about 2 cups) fresh shelled peas, blanched (see Tip, page 69) or frozen peas, thawed

½ teaspoon coarse kosher salt plus more to taste

1 pound best-quality dried tagliatelle or other flat, wide pasta such as fettuccine

1 tablespoon finely grated lemon zest

2 tablespoons finely chopped fresh tarragon plus sprigs to garnish if desired

Before You Start Availability of fresh morels is highly seasonal, but dried morels make a very good substitute and are usually available year-round in specialty food stores and gourmet food markets (or see Sources, page 273). If you can't find fresh or dried morels, you can substitute eight ounces of quartered cremini mushrooms. The dish will not reach quite the same depth of flavor but will be good nonetheless. Add the mushrooms with a tablespoon of butter to the pan after the shallots are softened, cook for 5–7 minutes until the mushrooms are golden, and then proceed with the recipe as written.

1. If using dried morsels, soak them in warm water for 15–20 minutes to soften. Rinse them thoroughly, squeeze them dry, and coarsely chop them.

2. Put a large pot of salted water on to boil for the pasta. In a small saucepan set over medium heat, heat the olive oil until hot. Add the shallots and cook, stirring occasionally, for 3–4 minutes until they are soft but not colored.

3. Add the white wine to the pan and increase the heat to medium-high. Bring to a simmer and simmer until reduced by half, about 4–5 minutes.

¼ cup crème fraîche (optional, see Tip below)

Freshly ground black pepper to taste

4. Reduce the heat under the sauce to medium and add the cream and morels to the pan. Bring to a gentle simmer and cook, uncovered, for 10 minutes. Add the peas and salt to the sauce and simmer for another 5 minutes to warm the peas. Remove the pan from the heat and cover.

5. While the sauce is simmering, cook the pasta according to the package directions.

6. Put the lemon zest, chopped tarragon, and crème fraîche, if using, in a large serving bowl.

7. When the pasta is cooked, drain it and immediately put it in the serving bowl. Pour the warm sauce over the pasta and toss to combine well. Adjust seasoning to taste. Serve immediately, garnished with sprigs of fresh tarragon if desired.

Tip: *Crème fraîche can be found in specialty food stores and well-stocked supermarkets, but you can also make it at home if you like. We have had best success with pasteurized (not ultrapasteurized) cream. In a small saucepan, gently warm 1 cup of heavy cream to about 100°F or until it feels warm to the touch, 5–7 minutes. Pour the mixture into a clean glass jar, stir in 2 tablespoons of buttermilk, and let stand in a warm place, loosely covered, until thickened, which can take as little as 8 hours or up to 36. Cover tightly and refrigerate for up to a week.*

A Vermont Spring Tonic: Rhubarb-Citrus Soda

As soon as the ground thawed in the spring, early settlers followed the example of native peoples and went digging for roots, where the concentrated energy of the plant had receded during the long winter. They crushed the roots and brewed invigorating teas and tonics, including the classic root beer. Although this recipe does not use roots, it does star one of spring's first home-garden harvests: rosy pink stalks of rhubarb unfurling themselves into the warming air. I learned this honey-sweetened natural soda technique from Ferrisburgh's Honey Gardens Apiaries, from which the Inn buys some of its honey. ◇ ***Makes: 1 gallon***

4 cups (about 1 pound) chopped rhubarb

2 quarts water

1 cup freshly squeezed orange juice (see Tip, page 75)

½ cup freshly squeezed lemon juice

1 cup honey plus more to taste

2 quarts plain seltzer, chilled

Before You Start   Use pink (not green) rhubarb for the most gorgeous sunrise shade. The tonic also makes an elegant base for a sparkling white wine cocktail.

1. Put the rhubarb and water into a large pot set over high heat. Cover the pot and bring it to a boil. Reduce the heat and simmer, covered, for about 20 minutes.

2. Pour the orange and lemon juices and honey into a 3-quart or larger container. Pour the hot rhubarb through a strainer into the container, pressing on the rhubarb to release all the flavor. Discard the rhubarb.

3. Whisk to dissolve the honey in the warm liquid. Taste and add more honey if desired, keeping in mind that you will be diluting the base with seltzer.

4. Cool to room temperature and then refrigerate in a sealed container. When ready to use, pour some of the rhubarb base into a glass and add seltzer in roughly equal parts to achieve the desired flavor and carbonation level. The base should keep in the refrigerator for up to a month.

Variation There is no end to the creative fruit soda combinations you can make. Honey Gardens suggests making mint-lime soda with 15–20 sprigs of fresh mint steeped for at least 45 minutes in 2 quarts of boiling water and then strained. Stir in 1 cup of honey and the juice of 7 limes and 1 lemon. For a spicy, Jamaican-style ginger ale, bring 2 quarts of water to a boil and add 1½ cups grated ginger root. Simmer, covered, for 20–30 minutes. Take the pot off the heat and add 1 cup of honey and the juice of 1 lemon and 1 lime. Let the mixture sit for at least 30 minutes and up to 5 hours, and then strain out the ginger root.

Tip: *To get the most juice from a citrus fruit, have the fruit at room temperature (or microwave it for a few seconds) and then roll it hard against the counter a few times before squeezing.*

Rhubarb and Yogurt Fool

This makes a beautiful and elegant springtime dessert served in small glass bowls and paired with another iconic Vermont spring ingredient, represented by a Maple Gingersnaps (page 262) or a few shards of Maple-Almond Brittle (page 270) perched on top. ◇ *Serves: 4*

6 cups (about 1½ pounds) chopped rhubarb

1 generous teaspoon freshly grated ginger

2 tablespoons orange liqueur, such as Grand Marnier

⅔ cup honey

1 cup best quality plain yogurt, preferably not nonfat

Before You Start Again, you will want the pink or red-tinted rhubarb, not the green variety. Fools are traditionally made with whipped cream instead of yogurt. Whipped cream is a perfectly fine option, but we like the lighter and tangier yogurt.

1. Preheat the oven to 350°F. Put the rhubarb in a 9 by 13-inch or other shallow 3-quart baking dish. Toss in the ginger and orange liqueur. Drizzle the honey over the rhubarb.

2. Bake uncovered for about 30 minutes until the rhubarb is completely soft. Cool for about 10 minutes.

3. Using a slotted spoon, spoon the rhubarb into the bowl of a food processor or into a blender. Add 3 tablespoons of the cooking liquid and puree until smooth.

4. For each serving, fold about ¼ cup yogurt into ½ cup of rhubarb puree and drizzle more of the cooking liquid over the top.

Variation This recipe would also work well with plums, apricots, or peaches, in which case you will need about 2 pounds of fruit to account for the pits and you can cut the honey down to ¼ cup. Cut the stone fruits in half and discard the pits. When they are cooked and cooled, the flesh should pull away fairly easily from the skins, which can be discarded before you puree the fruit—or this would be a great place to use a food mill.

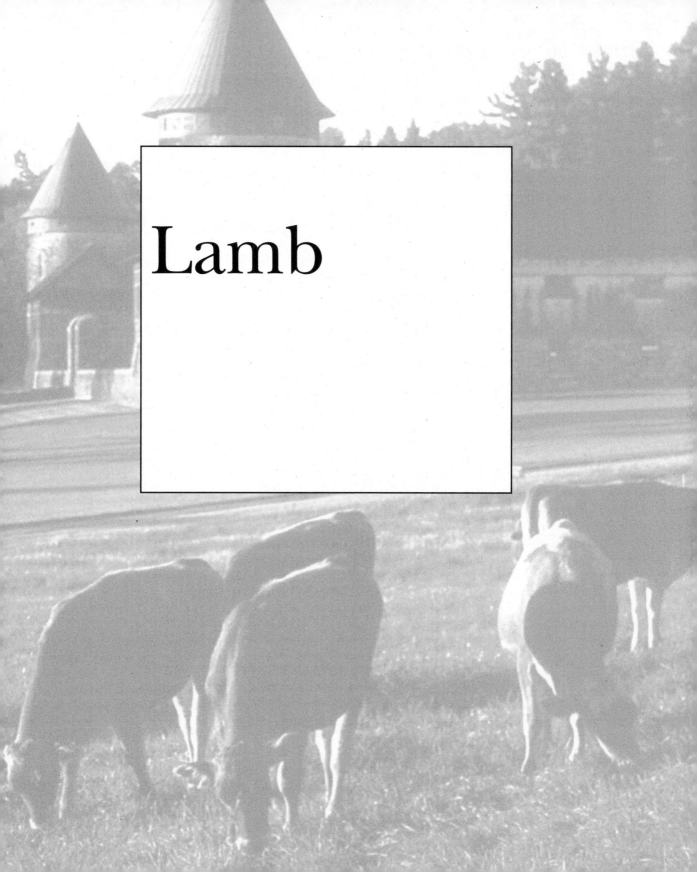

Lamb

- Braised Lamb with New Peas, Dill, and Sour Cream
- Lamb Shanks with Wheat Berries and Parsnips
- Lamb Sausage and Lentils
- Lamb, Red Onion, and Lemon Skewers on Grilled Bread Salad
- Spice-Rubbed Lamb Chops with Fennel, Chickpeas, and Tomatoes
- Lamb Burgers with Red Pepper and Black Olive Relish
- Smoke-Grilled Leg of Lamb with Eggplant and Tomato Salad
- Lamb and Fennel Bolognese
- Roasted Lamb Shoulder with Lemony New Potatoes
- Shepherd's Pie with Caramelized Onions and Cheddar Smash

*t*welve-year-old Jaba is king of the Children's Farmyard. The grizzled Romney ram plants himself solidly between the two indoor pens that are home to the Shelburne Farms breeding flock from late fall into spring. Like a big (but not exactly fierce) watchdog, the sheep patriarch lies in the middle of the path, staking out his territory and watching over the pregnant ewes. He has sired many lambs himself and has even mustered a few surprise offspring recently, says farmer Sam Smith with a smile as he digs his hand deep into Jaba's thick coat to give him a scratch.

Despite folklore to the contrary, cows have never actually outnumbered people in Vermont—but sheep have. From the 1820s to the 1860s, Vermont farmers jumped wholeheartedly into the business of raising wool to satisfy the booming New England textile mills, bringing the sheep population at one point to well over one and a half million animals against a human count of less than three hundred thousand. Lamb and mutton for the farmhouse table were an inevitable sideline, and spring lamb was especially welcomed as the first fresh meat after a long winter. But prices fell and the frontier pushed westward, opening up the wide, flat plains of the Midwest, a more economical place to raise sheep than hilly, rocky Vermont.

When the Webbs founded Shelburne Farms, Seward Webb did his part to keep sheep farming going in Vermont, maintaining a flock of between one hundred and two hundred purebred English sheep and making ram lambs available to other farms. He was particularly proud of his purebred Shropshire and Southdown sheep, which were raised to provide lamb and mutton for the family table. In 1941, Seward's grandson Derick started up sheep farming again with a flock of Shropshire mixes and sold the lamb to a high-end food market in Burlington.

The current flock of sheep on Shelburne Farms includes Texels with white faces and black noses and Tunis with caramel-colored faces and floppy ears. Of the fifty sheep, about thirty-five ewes are bred every fall to lamb in the late winter and early spring. They are shorn right before going out to pasture in April, and the wool is sold at the Welcome Center. The sheep are raised largely on pasture and provide meat for the Inn's restaurant, where lamb is simmered into a rich Bolognese, cured into prosciutto, slow-roasted and topped with fried mint, or encrusted with black olives and feta and seared until just rosy pink.

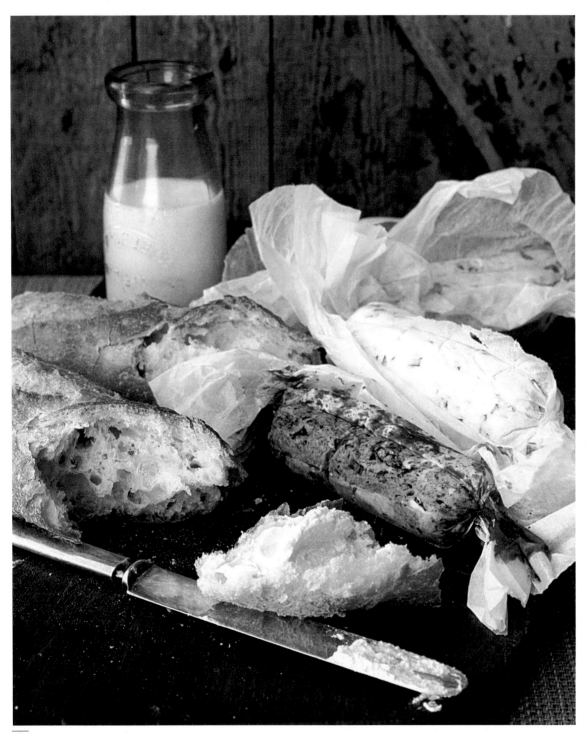

Home-Churned Butter *(page 6)* and Compound Butters (from top):
Orange-Rosemary, Mint-Lemon, and Red Wine-Shallot *(pages 10, 9, and 10)*

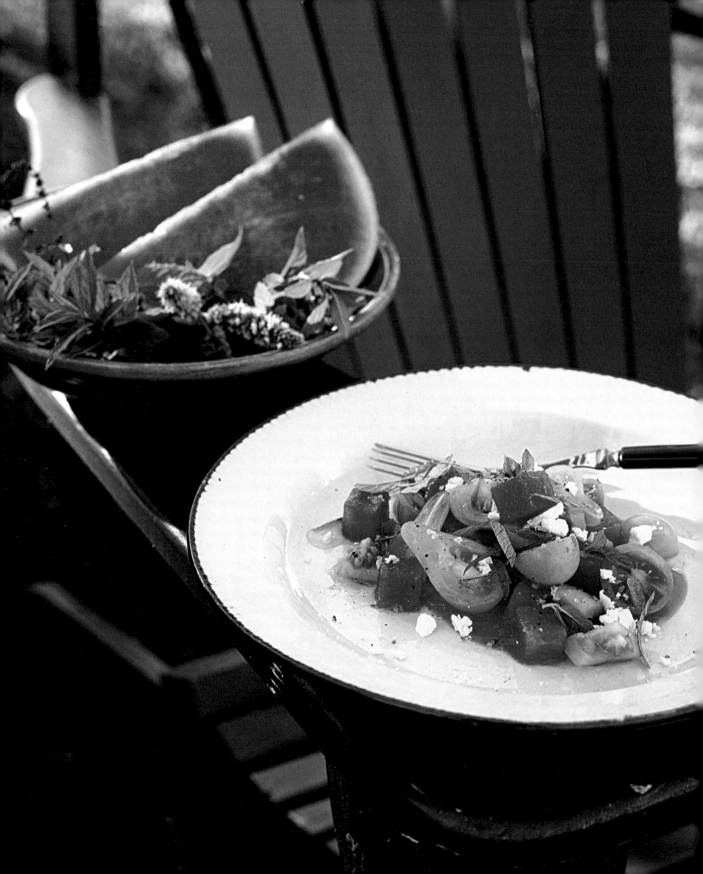

Green Mountain
Ploughman's Lunch
(page 21) with Inn at
Shelburne Farms
Pickled Ramps
(page 59) and Apple-
Rhubarb Chutney
(page 215)

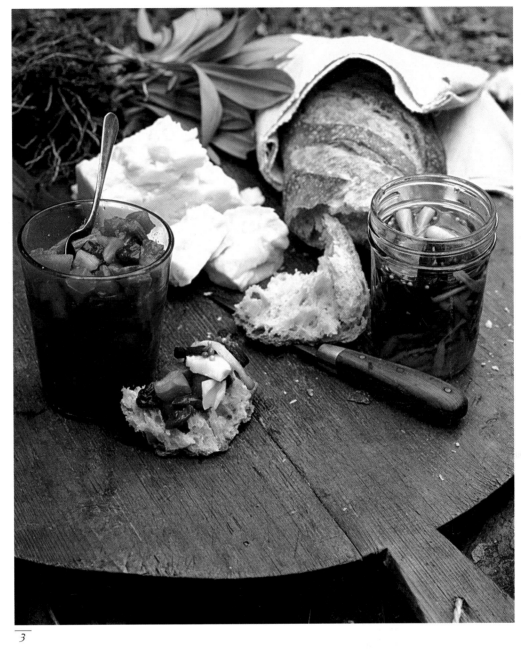

3

Opposite: Watermelon, Tomato,
and Feta Salad *(page 17)*

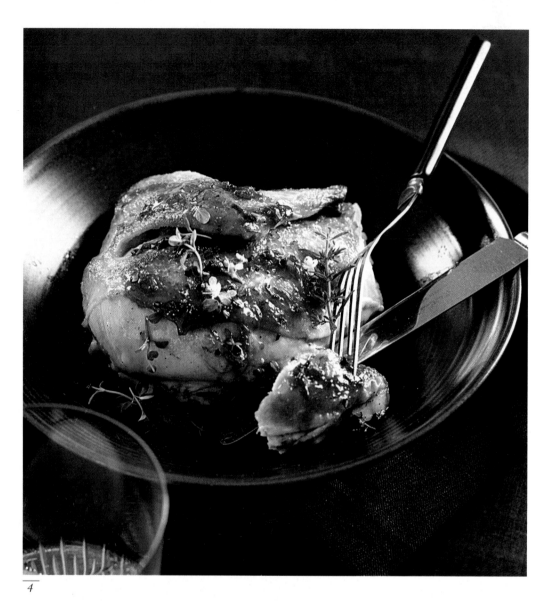

Maple and Black Pepper Chicken *(page 48)*

Opposite: Springtime Eggs Benedict with
Wild Greens and Mushrooms *(page 57)*

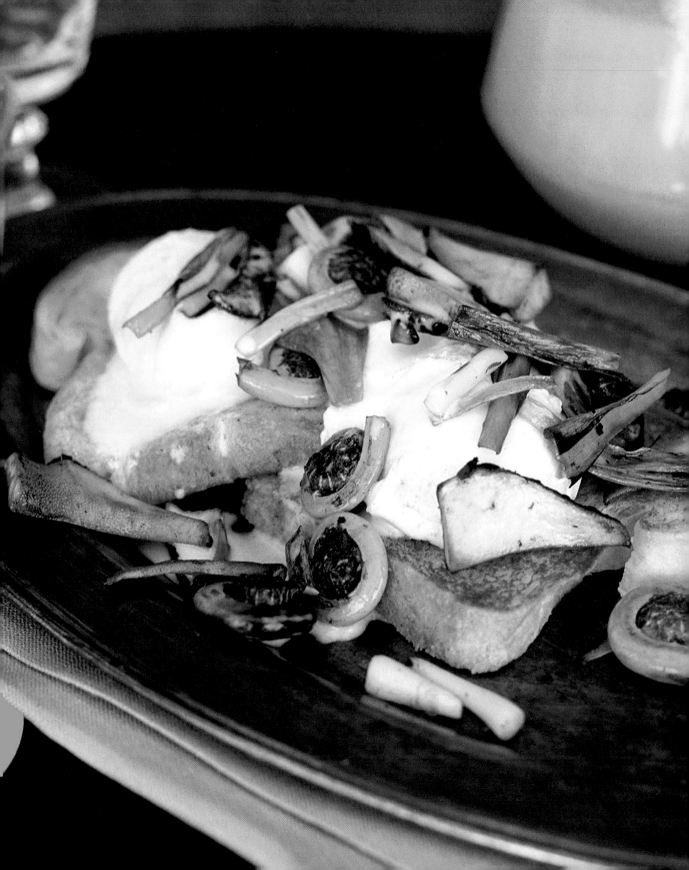

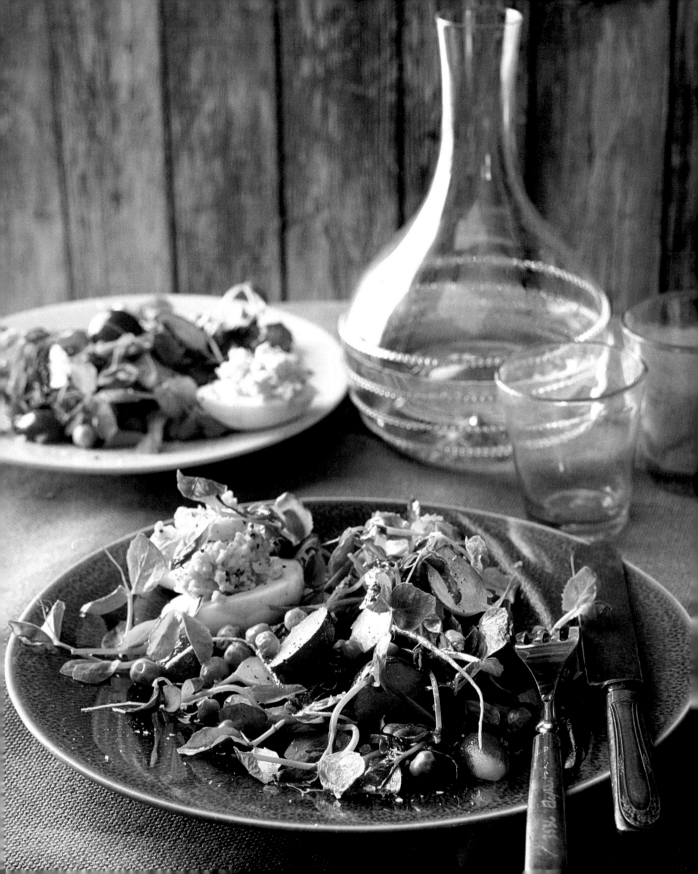

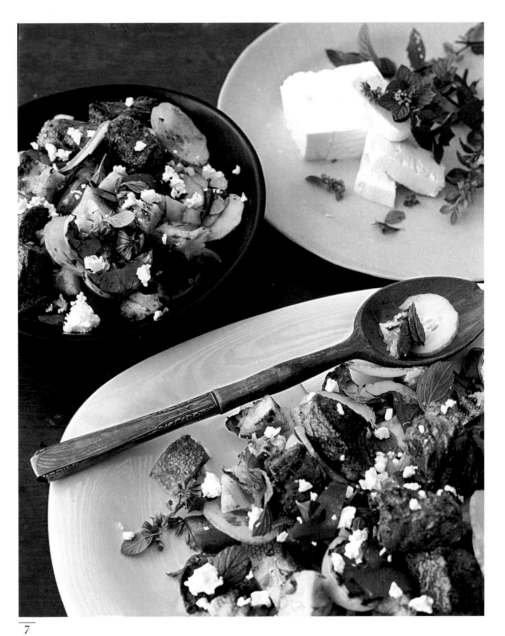

Lamb, Red Onion,
and Lemon Skewers
on Grilled Bread
Salad *(page 90)*

Opposite: The Whole-Pea Salad with
Deviled Farm Barn Eggs
(page 68)

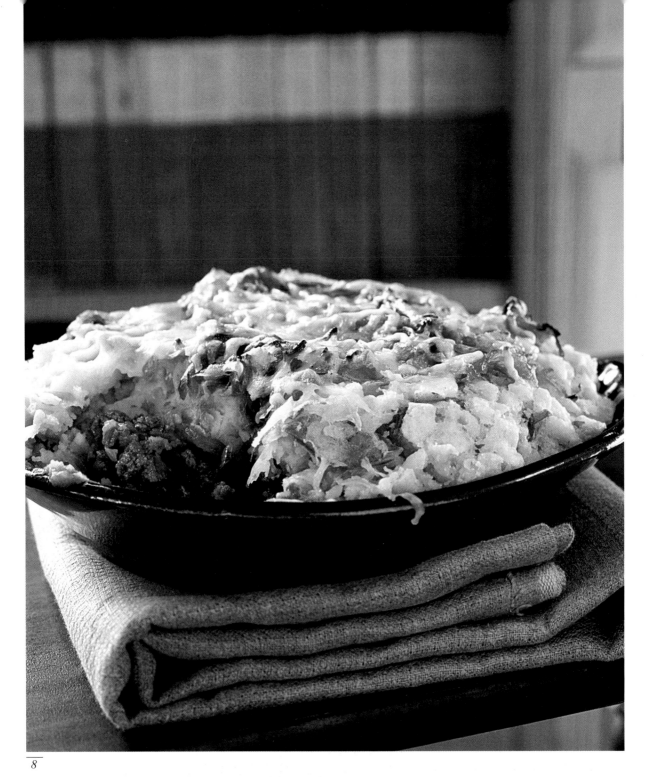

Shepherd's Pie with Caramelized Onions and
Cheddar Smash *(page 99)*

A Note on Lamb

There is more to lamb than tiny, tender loin chops and succulent roasted leg with mint sauce. We love those too, but at the Inn, Rick gets the whole lambs that have grown on the surrounding pasture and he challenges himself to use as much of the animal as possible. "My mission is not to throw any of it away," he says, which means he spends time really thinking about ways to use the less commonly seen parts of the animal and, occasionally, explaining to diners why he doesn't offer full rack of lamb. ("I'd only have enough for one night a week," he says.) The results of his creativity range from his very popular lamb sliders, upon which we based our Lamb Burgers (page 93), to delicious morsels of fried lamb's tongue on the charcuterie platter (let us know if you want that recipe).

We recommend searching out local lamb that has been raised on pasture. Although people often think of lamb at two ends of a spectrum—either very delicate or quite strong and gamy—most lamb raised today has sweet, earthy, and light gamy notes. If the flavors are too strong, most likely the lamb is not as fresh as it should be.

We have found that ground lamb is especially variable, and because it will often have a fairly high level of fat, it can develop strong flavors. If you have access to a good butcher counter, it is always best to ask for your lamb to be ground fresh to order. The leanest (and priciest) ground lamb will be from the leg, but a well-trimmed shoulder is often your best bet. Good ground lamb can also come from the neck or a well-trimmed breast.

Grilled or roasted lamb is always best cooked just until medium-rare or to an internal temperature of not more than 145°F after resting. For larger pieces of lamb, like roasts, that means you will want to pull them off the heat at closer to 140°F, as the temperature of the meat will continue to rise when the meat juices redistribute themselves during resting.

Lamb

Braised Lamb with New Peas, Dill, and Sour Cream

A classic Scandinavian flavor combination with a lovely, light spring feeling. Serve it over noodles or mashed potatoes. ◇ *Serves: 4–6*

⅓ cup all-purpose flour

1½ teaspoons coarse kosher salt plus more to taste

1½ pounds lamb stew meat (see Before You Start), cut into 1½-inch pieces

3–4 tablespoons olive oil

1 medium onion, halved and thinly sliced crosswise

1 cup dry white wine

2 cups chicken stock, preferably low sodium

2 cups small fresh peas (blanched first if not tiny and tender; see Tip, page 69) or frozen peas, thawed

2 tablespoons chopped fresh dill plus additional for garnish

½ cup sour cream, not nonfat

1 teaspoon lemon zest

1–2 teaspoons freshly squeezed lemon juice

Freshly ground black pepper to taste

Before You Start   With prepackaged lamb stew meat, it's often hard to tell what you're getting; we like well-trimmed shoulder best here, but stew meat cut from the breast will work too.

1. Pour the flour into a shallow, rimmed plate or pie pan and whisk in 1 teaspoon of the salt. Pat the lamb dry and dredge it lightly in the flour mixture.

2. In a large sauté pan or skillet set over medium-high heat, heat 2 tablespoons of the olive oil. When the oil is hot, brown the lamb, in batches if necessary so as not to crowd the pan, adding more olive oil as needed. Cook without moving the meat until a nice golden brown crust develops, 2–3 minutes on each side. Remove the lamb to a plate.

3. Add the remaining tablespoon of olive oil to the pan, and then add the onion. Cook, stirring occasionally, for 2–3 minutes or until the onion has softened and colored. Add the white wine and deglaze the pan, stirring to scrape up any brown bits. Simmer for 2–3 minutes. Add the lamb and any accumulated juices back to the pan. Add the chicken stock and bring to a simmer. Cover the pot with a lid slightly ajar and maintain a gentle simmer for 45 minutes to 1 hour until the lamb is tender.

4. Stir in the peas and bring the pot back up to a simmer for 5 minutes, or until the peas are cooked. Reduce the heat to medium-low and stir in the chopped dill, sour cream, lemon zest, 1 teaspoon of the lemon juice, and the remaining ½ teaspoon of salt. Do not allow to boil.

5. Warm through for 4–5 minutes, adjust seasoning to taste, and add more lemon juice to taste. Serve garnished with additional fresh dill if desired.

Lamb

Lamb Shanks with Wheat Berries and Parsnips

Here is an ode to an underappreciated trio: lamb shanks, deeply delicious but a bit off-putting if you're new to them; nutty and pleasantly chewy wheat berries, which are simply unhulled kernels of wheat; and parsnips, sweet, pale cousin to the carrot. This slow-cooked dish is perfect mid-winter Vermont fare. ◇ *Serves: 4–6*

1½ cups hard, red wheat berries, soaked overnight in water

2 sprigs fresh rosemary

6 sprigs fresh thyme

1 bay leaf

4 lamb shanks, about 1 pound each

1 teaspoon coarse kosher salt plus more to taste

Freshly ground black pepper to taste

2 tablespoons olive oil

2 large carrots (about ½ pound), peeled and cut into 1-inch pieces

2 medium parsnips (about ½ pound), peeled and cut into 1-inch pieces

1 medium onion, peeled and cut into 1-inch chunks

1 large celery stalk, coarsely chopped

4 garlic cloves, smashed with the flat side of a knife and peeled

1½ cups dry red wine

1 (14½-ounce) can diced tomatoes with their juice

2 cups chicken stock, preferably low sodium

Before You Start We have found that some wheat berries (probably because of age) can benefit from an overnight soak to soften their hull and speed up cooking. Since you won't know the age of yours, it's a safe step to take. We are lucky to be able to find them grown locally in northern Vermont, but they are also available in the bulk bins of natural foods stores nationwide. If you cannot find wheat berries, substitute unsoaked but rinsed pearl barley and skip the twenty minutes of simmering on the stove because the quicker-cooking barley will have plenty of time in the oven. Be forewarned that the barley will turn an interesting shade of purple thanks to the red wine.

1. The night before you will be cooking, put the wheat berries in a large bowl and cover them with cold water.

2. Tie the rosemary, thyme, and bay leaf up in a cheesecloth bag and set aside. Pat the lamb shanks dry and season them with the salt and pepper to taste.

3. In a large Dutch oven set over medium-high heat, heat 1 tablespoon of the olive oil. When the oil is hot, brown the shanks, in batches if necessary so as not to crowd the pan. Cook, turning periodically, until a nice crust has formed, about 8–10 minutes total. Remove the browned shanks to a plate.

4. Add the remaining tablespoon of olive oil to the pan and add the carrots, parsnips, onion, celery, and garlic cloves. Cook, stirring, for 7–9 minutes until the vegetables are turning golden. Add the wine and deglaze the pan, stirring to scrape up any brown bits. Simmer 5 minutes and then add the herb bundle, tomatoes with their juice, and chicken stock to the pan along with the drained wheat berries. Bring the pot to a simmer and cover. Simmer on the stove for 20 minutes.

5. While the wheat berries are simmering, preheat the oven to 350°F. Return the lamb shanks and any accumulated juices to the pot. Put the covered pot in the oven and cook for 1½–2 hours until the lamb and wheat berries are tender (the wheat berries will still have a little bite to them).

6. To serve, it is easiest to shred the meat off the bone in the kitchen and serve plates of wheat berries and vegetables topped with the shredded meat and cooking liquid.

> **Prepare-Ahead Tip:** *This dish is even better made the day ahead. Cool to room temperature and then chill, covered, in the refrigerator. Scrape any fat off the top before warming, covered, in a 350°F oven for 30–40 minutes.*

Lamb

Caring for the Flock

Sam Smith, farmer and educator,
Shelburne Farms

"I think the farmyard is probably the best place in the world to educate people about what they're eating."

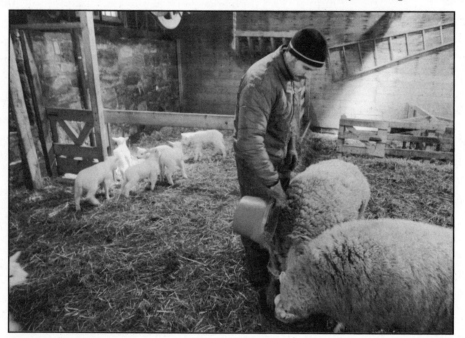

"ello, sheep!" says a very small visitor as she picks up some hay and shoves it through the gate of the winter Children's Farmyard pen. Thirty ewes turn mildly curious eyes toward the activity, but they soon see that it's not a real food delivery and return to chewing their cud and finding warmth hunkered down by the walls of the enclosure.

A few steps away in the Farmyard's education center, paddocks and bales of hay have temporarily replaced picture books and activity posters. The first few lambs of the season stick close to their mothers as sparrows swoop down from the eaves to peck at the floor and perch on the edges of frosty water buckets. The youngest, just forty-eight hours old and covered in cocoa-brown, nappy wool, is curled under the protective shelter of his mother's chin. "Tunis are good mothers," Sam says with approval.

The ewe he expects to deliver next is in the pen with the lambs. She is also a Tunis, and her name is Rita. When she is lying down, you can see movement under her wooly side, as if a wave is swelling within her. "She's still chewing her cud, though," Sam observes, "so she's probably not going yet." He's not worried, because she's an experienced mother: "The old ewes know how to do it," he says.

Sam did not grow up with livestock, but he seems comfortable with lambing and jokes easily about being the expectant dad for more than thirty-five newborn sheep. Before coming to Shelburne Farms, he worked as a vegetable farmer and as a case manager for homeless teens. All jobs have their challenges, he acknowledges, "but the worries are a lot different." Over the last few years, he has worked closely with colleagues at the Farm, sheep experts at the University of Vermont, and the Farm's longtime veterinarian. He tries to let the ewes give birth with as little interference as possible. "A normal birth," he says with awe in his voice, "is gorgeous." But he'll pull up his sleeves, slather on the disinfectant, and reach in if need be.

The Shelburne Farms' Children's Farmyard is an educational farm within the working farm, where visitors can milk a cow or goat, collect eggs, and learn how to carefully pick up a chicken, feed the animals, and maybe even witness a sow or a ewe giving birth. The natural cycle of a farm also, undeniably, includes the other end of life. A poster on the wall of the Farmyard carefully explains the life of a Shelburne Farms lamb and finishes with a photograph of a beautifully plated dish from the Inn. It is true that lambs are about as cute as food gets, and that makes some people uncomfortable, but "we raise animals for human consumption here," Sam says plainly. "People need to recognize where their food is coming from."

It is most important to Sam—and to Shelburne Farms—that the flock be managed to the highest environmental and humane standards, leaving the animals on pasture and the lambs with their mothers as long as possible. "I raise them in the best way that I can, and I try to educate people," he says. "You can't force people to do anything, but you can educate them. And I think the farmyard is probably the best place in the world to educate people about what they're eating."

Lamb Sausage and Lentils

In the fall, Rick offers a cassoulet made with slow-cooked beans and Merguez sausage, a traditional North African lamb sausage spiced with red chili paste. We sped it up by using nutty, little green lentils. It is not a beautiful dish, but the golden shards of rosemary-scented bread have their own rustic charm, and the flavors are deep and woodsy with a good kick from the sausage. ◇ **Serves: 4–6**

2 cups (about ¾ pound) small French green lentils (see Before You Start), rinsed and picked over for stones or other seeds

6 cups water

1 teaspoon coarse kosher salt plus more to taste

2 sprigs fresh rosemary plus 2 teaspoons finely minced rosemary

1 pound lamb sausage, such as Merguez (see Before You Start)

3 tablespoons olive oil

2 medium leeks, white and light green parts only, halved lengthwise, thinly sliced, and rinsed thoroughly

1 tablespoon stone-ground mustard plus more to taste

2 tablespoons cider vinegar

Freshly ground black pepper to taste

4 thick slices crusty, country-style bread, chopped into coarse crumbs (about 4 cups)

Before You Start   Lentilles du Puy, the tiny green lentils originally from Puy, France, are more delicate and hold their shape better than the larger brown lentils. They can be found in natural or specialty foods stores and are worth searching out. Merguez sausage seems to be the most consistently flavored and widely available type of lamb sausage; most butchers can order it if they don't stock it (see Sources, page 273). In Vermont, we are able to buy good local lamb sausage made with sage and garlic, which works very well in this recipe. If you can find a nicely flavored, locally made sausage (skip any with strong flavors like mint), feel free to use that. You could also use similarly seasoned turkey or chicken sausage in this recipe.

1. In a large saucepan set over medium-high heat, place the lentils with the water, salt, and rosemary sprigs. Cover and bring the pot to a boil. Reduce the heat to simmer, covered, for 20–25 minutes until the lentils are just tender. (They will cook a little more in the oven.) Before draining the lentils, scoop out ½ cup of the cooking liquid and reserve.

2. While the lentils are cooking, preheat the oven to 400°F and set a rack in the second-highest slot. Split the sausages down the middle lengthwise and remove the meat from the casings. Discard the casings.

3. In a large sauté pan or skillet set over medium-high heat, heat 1 teaspoon of the olive oil. Add the lamb sausage and cook, stirring occasionally, until it starts to color, 4–5 minutes.

4. Discard all but 1 tablespoon of the fat in the pan and add the leeks. Continue cooking, stirring occasionally, until the sausage is browned and the leeks are golden, another 5 minutes.

5. Distribute the drained lentils evenly into a shallow 2- or 3-quart baking dish. Add the sausage and leeks, mustard, and cider vinegar. Stir to combine, adding the reserved lentil cooking liquid to moisten. Adjust seasoning and add more mustard to taste.

6. Toss the bread with the remaining olive oil and the minced rosemary. Strew over the top of the lentils and sausage. Bake for 20 minutes until the bread crumbs are crisp and golden. Serve immediately.

Lamb, Red Onion, and Lemon Skewers on Grilled Bread Salad

[photograph 7]

The kiss of fire on the lamb, lemon, and bread really add to this summery grill recipe. It has a few different parts, but the sum of the whole is a company-worthy, all-in-one meal. You could try it in the broiler, but we think it's really worth waiting for grill season. ◇ **Serves: 6**

For the lamb

2 tablespoons plain yogurt

1 tablespoon finely chopped fresh oregano

1 tablespoon finely chopped fresh mint

¾ teaspoon ground cumin

½ teaspoon garam masala (see Before You Start)

1½ teaspoons coarse kosher salt plus more to taste

2 cloves garlic, minced

2 teaspoons freshly squeezed lemon juice

1½ pounds boneless leg of lamb, trimmed and cut into 2-inch cubes

For the skewers and salad

1 red onion, cut into 8 wedges, each cut in half crosswise

1 thin-skinned lemon, scrubbed well and cut into 8 wedges, each cut in half crosswise (see Before You Start)

3 tablespoons olive oil

Before You Start This dish requires a little advance planning, as the lamb needs to marinate for at least two hours. Also, if you're going to use bamboo skewers, soak them in water for at least thirty minutes before grilling. Garam masala is an Indian spice mixture with hints of cinnamon, chili, mace, and coriander. It can be found in Indian groceries and some well-stocked supermarkets. It is critical to use thin-skinned lemons, such as Meyer, or the bitter pith can overwhelm the dish. Pick lemons with the most give when you squeeze them, an indication that they probably have skin less than ⅛-inch thick.

1. ***Marinate the lamb:*** In a medium bowl, whisk together the yogurt, oregano, mint, cumin, garam masala, salt, garlic, and lemon juice. Toss the lamb cubes in the marinade, cover, and refrigerate for at least 2 hours but not more than 24.

2. ***Make the skewers and salad:*** Prepare a barbecue grill to cook on medium-high heat. Remove the lamb from the marinade. On each skewer, thread a few cubes of lamb alternately with bite-size chunks of onion and at least one lemon piece with the rind facing out so it will be exposed to the grill heat. Drizzle the skewers with 1 tablespoon of the olive oil and season with a little salt and pepper. Brush the bread slices on both sides with another tablespoon of the olive oil and season with salt and pepper to taste.

Coarse kosher salt to taste

Freshly ground black pepper to taste

4 slices crusty, country-style bread, about ¾ inch thick

½ cup coarsely chopped fresh mint

½ cup (2–3 ounces) crumbled feta

½ long English cucumber, thinly sliced and unpeeled, or 1 regular cucumber, peeled, seeded, and thinly sliced

3. Grill the skewers, turning occasionally, until the onion has softened, the lemons are lightly charred, and the lamb is medium-rare—about 10 minutes. Grill the bread about 2 minutes per side until golden brown.

4. Carefully pull the lamb, onion, and lemon off the skewers into separate piles. Coarsely chop the onions and place them in a large mixing bowl. Add the mint, feta, and cucumber.

5. Cut the grilled bread into 1-inch cubes and add to the bowl. Finely chop about half the charred lemon pieces to measure ¼ cup and add to the bowl. (Reserve the remaining charred lemon pieces for garnish.)

6. Drizzle the salad with the remaining tablespoon of olive oil and mix to combine all the ingredients (hands work well here). Season to taste with salt and pepper. Mound the salad onto a serving platter and top with the lamb. Garnish with the remaining charred lemon pieces and serve.

Prepare-Ahead Tip: *This dish can be prepared two or three hours ahead through step 4. Keep the lamb, onion, lemons, and salad in the refrigerator and the bread at room temperature. Bring everything to room temperature before serving.*

Spice-Rubbed Lamb Chops with Fennel, Chickpeas, and Tomatoes

These lamb chops and salad have an exotic Middle Eastern inflection, with the cardamom adding a slightly mysterious and alluring flavor. ◇ *Serves: 4*

For the lamb chops

1½ teaspoons ground cardamom

1 tablespoon ground cumin

2 teaspoons coarse kosher salt plus more to taste

1½ teaspoons freshly ground black pepper

8 lamb loin or rib chops (1-inch thick, about 3 pounds total)

For the salad

½ cup plain yogurt

1 teaspoon cumin

1 teaspoon coarse kosher salt

2 teaspoons freshly squeezed lemon juice

2 tablespoons olive oil

2 small fennel bulbs or one large bulb (about 1 pound with stalks)

1 (15-ounce) can chickpeas (garbanzo beans), drained and rinsed

2 large red tomatoes (about 1 pound total), cored and cut into bite-size chunks

⅓ cup coarsely chopped fresh flat-leaf parsley

Before You Start   The fennel should be sliced very thin with a mandoline-type slicer or a very sharp knife.

1. Prepare a barbecue grill to cook on medium-high heat. Alternatively, place a large broiler-proof skillet, preferably cast iron, on an oven rack set in the second-highest position, about 4–5 inches from the heating element. Preheat the broiler on its highest setting for at least 15 minutes.

2. *Prepare the lamb chops:* In a small bowl, whisk together the cardamom, cumin, salt, and pepper. Rub the mixture over the lamb chops and set them aside while preparing the salad.

3. *Prepare the salad:* In a large serving bowl, whisk together the yogurt, cumin, salt, lemon juice, and olive oil. Trim the fennel of stalks and tough part of the core. Cut in half from the top to the root lengthwise. Shave or slice very thinly crosswise.

4. Place the fennel, chickpeas, tomato, and parsley in the bowl with the dressing and toss gently to coat. Adjust seasoning to taste. Set aside.

5. Grill or broil the lamb chops to desired doneness, about 5 minutes per side for medium-rare. Let rest for 4–5 minutes before serving with the salad.

Lamb Burgers with Red Pepper and Black Olive Relish

At the Inn, Rick offers mini versions of these as an appetizer on little challah rolls with grilled red pepper relish and black olive aioli. We streamlined and folded the black olives into the relish. Serve the burgers on really good soft buns, lightly grilled. ◇ *Serves: 4*

For the relish

2 medium red bell peppers, grilled or broiled until charred and then skinned, seeded, and coarsely chopped (see Tip below)

⅓ cup coarsely chopped, pitted, vinegar-marinated black olives, such as kalamata

¼ cup coarsely chopped fresh flat-leaf parsley

2 teaspoons freshly squeezed lemon juice

2 tablespoons extra-virgin olive oil

Coarse kosher salt to taste

For the burgers

1½ pounds lean ground lamb

¼ cup finely chopped fresh flat-leaf parsley

½ teaspoon crushed red pepper

1 tablespoon finely minced garlic

1 teaspoon coarse kosher salt

1 teaspoon freshly ground black pepper

Before You Start See A Note on Lamb (page 83) for tips on buying ground lamb. We allow for a 6-ounce burger because even lean ground lamb will shrink quite a bit on the grill. If you don't have time to grill or broil the peppers yourself, the jarred roasted red peppers often found in the Italian sections of well-stocked supermarkets make a fine substitute; just make sure not to buy the marinated kind and to pat them dry before using. If you can't cook the burgers on a grill, use a good, heavy frying pan, preferably a ridged grill pan, on the stove; lamb burgers can cause dangerous flare-ups in a broiler.

1. Prepare a barbecue grill to cook on medium-high heat.

2. Prepare the relish: In a small serving bowl, stir together the peppers, olives, parsley, lemon juice, olive oil, and salt.

3. Prepare the burgers: In a large bowl, mix together the ground lamb, parsley, red pepper, garlic, salt, and black pepper. Form the mixture into four burgers, flatten them to about ¾ inch thick, and gently press your thumb in the center of each one to help them cook evenly.

4. Grill or panfry the burgers carefully for about 3–4 minutes per side for medium-rare. (Be forewarned that the fat in lamb can cause flare-ups.) Serve the burgers topped with the relish.

> ***Tip:*** *After grilling or broiling the peppers, put them in a bowl and cover it tightly with plastic wrap. Leave the peppers for about 8–10 minutes and the skin will be much easier to remove.*

Smoke-Grilled Leg of Lamb with Eggplant and Tomato Salad

This dish makes a beautiful presentation with the pink lamb, dark purple–edged eggplant, and deep red tomatoes flecked with the green of fresh marjoram—it is perfect for a summer gathering. ◇ *Serves: 6–8*

1 butterflied leg of lamb, about 3½–4 pounds

3 large cloves garlic, finely chopped

2 tablespoons finely chopped fresh marjoram plus more for garnish as desired

3 tablespoons freshly squeezed lemon juice

½ cup plus 2 tablespoons olive oil

1 tablespoon coarse kosher salt plus more to taste

Freshly ground black pepper to taste

2 medium eggplants (about 1 pound each), cut lengthwise into ¾-inch-thick slices

6 plum tomatoes, cored

2 tablespoons capers, drained and rinsed

1 tablespoon red wine vinegar

Before You Start   We don't recommend trying this in the broiler; it just won't be the same. Marjoram is a sadly underused herb with a light, sweet, piney flavor that goes especially well with lamb. If you can't find fresh marjoram, use oregano instead.

1. Prepare a barbecue grill to cook on high heat. If you are using a gas grill, see the Tip on page 95. Lay the butterflied leg of lamb out flat and cut it into three roughly similar-size pieces for easier handling and more even cooking.

2. In a small bowl, whisk together the garlic, 1 tablespoon of the chopped marjoram, 2 tablespoons of the lemon juice, and ¼ cup of the olive oil. Rub the mixture liberally over the lamb, and then season the lamb with 2 teaspoons of the salt and ground pepper to taste on both sides. Let sit for at least 30 minutes or, in the refrigerator, not more than 12 hours.

3. Brush the eggplant slices and plum tomatoes with another ¼ cup of the olive oil and sprinkle with the remaining teaspoon of salt.

4. When the grill is hot, lay the lamb, eggplant, and tomatoes on the grill. You may not be able to fit all the eggplant the first time. In that case, just add the remaining slices when you take off the first batch of eggplant.

5. After about 4–5 minutes, check the lamb and vegetables and turn them if they are starting to char. After a total of 8–9 minutes, the eggplant will probably be ready to come off the grill. Add any remaining eggplant and continue turning the tomatoes until they are evenly blistered, up to 15 minutes.

6. Turn the lamb back to its first side when you take the eggplant off, and then cover the grill. Check the tomatoes and any remaining eggplant slices in another 3–4 minutes and remove or turn as necessary. Turn the lamb one more time for a total of about 20–25 minutes' grill time or until it registers about 140°F on an instant-read thermometer. (See A Note on Lamb on page 81, for information on cooked lamb temperatures.) It may get a little charred in places.

7. Allow the lamb to rest for at least 10 minutes while you prepare the vegetables. Cut the eggplant into ¾-inch cubes and coarsely chop the tomatoes. Toss the vegetables in a bowl with the capers, red wine vinegar, the remaining tablespoon of lemon juice, the remaining tablespoon of chopped marjoram, and the remaining 2 tablespoons olive oil. Adjust seasoning to taste.

8. Slice the lamb thinly crosswise and present on a platter around the eggplant and tomato salad, garnished with additional marjoram sprigs as desired.

> **Tip:** *Rick is a fan of Steven Raichlen's book* How to Grill *and suggests following his advice to create smoke if you're using a gas grill. Soak one cup of apple or maple wood chips in water for about an hour. Place the drained chips in the middle of a large sheet of heavy-duty foil. Bring two sides of the foil to the center and fold the edges together and over twice to make a seam. Do the same with the other two sides so that the chips are completely sealed. Poke about ten holes in the foil with a sharp knife. Put the pouch in a corner of the grill when you start it up. When it's hot, it will produce smoke.*

Lamb and Fennel Bolognese

This is a version of the classic Italian Bolognese sauce, enriched with ground lamb and sweetened with fennel. At the Inn, Rick serves a similar sauce over housemade ricotta gnocchi or quill-shaped garganelli topped with a little mint and shaved, aged sheep's milk cheese made in Vermont at Woodcock Farm in Weston (see Sources, page 273). ◇ **Serves: 4–6 over 1 pound of pasta**

1 sprig fresh rosemary

5 large fresh sage leaves

1 teaspoon olive oil

1 pound lean ground lamb

1½ teaspoons coarse kosher salt plus more to taste

1 medium onion, cut into ¼-inch dice (about 1 cup)

1 large carrot, peeled and cut into ¼-inch dice (about 1 cup)

1 small fennel bulb (about ½ pound with stalks), trimmed and cut into ¼-inch dice (about 1–1½ cups)

2 cloves minced garlic

1 cup whole milk

½ cup dry white wine

1 (28-ounce) can crushed tomatoes

¼ teaspoon crushed red pepper

Freshly ground black pepper to taste

Before You Start   See A Note on Lamb (page 81) for tips on buying ground lamb. This chunky sauce works well over a variety of pasta shapes. In the long, flat family of pastas, try pappardelle or tagliatelle, or go with a substantial shape like ziti or rigatoni.

1. Tie the rosemary and sage in a cheesecloth bundle or in a bouquet with kitchen twine. Set aside.

2. In a large sauté pan or skillet set over medium-high heat, heat the olive oil until hot. Add the ground lamb in chunks and cook without moving the meat until a nice golden brown crust develops, 4–6 minutes. Season the lamb with 1 teaspoon of the salt. Turn the lamb and brown the other side in the same way.

3. When the lamb is browned, drain off and discard all the fat and put the pan back over medium heat. Add the onion, carrot, fennel, and garlic to the pan. Cook, stirring to break the lamb into smaller pieces, until the onion and fennel are softened, 5–7 minutes.

4. Add the milk and increase the heat to medium-high. Simmer until the milk has almost evaporated, 5–7 minutes. Add the white wine and simmer for 10 minutes. Add the tomatoes, red pepper, and herb bundle, and bring the sauce back to a simmer.

5. Simmer very gently for 1 hour, uncovered. Remove the herbs and discard. Add the remaining ½ teaspoon of salt. Adjust seasoning to taste and serve over pasta.

Roasted Lamb Shoulder with Lemony New Potatoes

The shoulder roast has fallen out of favor, but we think it deserves another chance; rubbed with herbs and a zing of red pepper and served with crusty potatoes bathed in lemon. It has a little more flavor than a leg of lamb—along with a few more tough bits to cut around—and we think it's worth it. If you have any leftover lamb, use it in the Shepherd's Pie (page 99). ◇ ***Serves: 6–8***

1 boneless, rolled, tied lamb shoulder, about 3½–4 pounds

1 lemon, well washed

1 tablespoon chopped fresh rosemary plus 3 whole rosemary sprigs

1 tablespoon finely minced garlic plus 4 garlic cloves, smashed with the flat side of a knife

½ teaspoon crushed red pepper, finely minced (see Before You Start)

½ teaspoon freshly ground black pepper plus more to taste

1½ teaspoons coarse kosher salt plus more to taste

2 pounds new potatoes or small potatoes cut into 1-inch chunks

2 tablespoons olive oil

Before You Start   Ask your butcher for a well-trimmed, boneless, rolled shoulder roast. If you can't find a shoulder roast, a boneless, tied leg will work too. An instant-read meat thermometer is critical for this recipe. You will need a very sharp knife to mince the crushed red pepper; alternatively, whir it in a spice grinder or grind it with a mortar and pestle. If you prefer less lemon flavor, just squeeze the juice over the potatoes and leave out the lemon zest.

1. Preheat the oven to 300°F with a rack in the second-highest slot. Set the lamb shoulder in a roasting pan with enough room for the potatoes around the roast. Using a vegetable peeler, peel long strips of zest from the lemon, making sure to avoid the bitter white pith. Set the zest aside. Cut the lemon in half and squeeze the juice from one half all over the roast. Reserve the remaining lemon half.

2. In a small bowl, combine the chopped rosemary, minced garlic, red pepper, black pepper, and 1 teaspoon of the salt. Rub the mixture vigorously all over the lamb shoulder and put it in the oven.

Lamb

3. Allowing 35–40 minutes per pound, roast the lamb until about 1 hour is left to reach medium-rare (this will be about 1 hour in for a 3½-pound roast). In a large bowl, toss the potatoes with the juice from the reserved lemon half, reserved lemon zest strips, whole rosemary sprigs, smashed garlic cloves, remaining ½ teaspoon salt, and olive oil. Baste the lamb with any pan juices, and then distribute the potato mixture around the lamb.

4. After another hour of roasting, check the internal temperature of the lamb and continue cooking until an instant-read thermometer inserted in the center of the roast reads 140°F (see A Note on Lamb, page 81, for information about cooked lamb temperatures). Remove the roast from the pan and set it on a carving board to rest, loosely covered with foil. Increase the oven temperature to 450°F and roast the potatoes for another 15–20 minutes until crusty.

5. Cut the twine from the lamb and carve slices to serve with the potatoes.

Shepherd's Pie with Caramelized Onions and Cheddar Smash

[photograph 8]

A true shepherd's pie is always made with lamb; the similar dish made with beef is properly called a cottage pie. It is one of the most comforting and homey dishes around. Traditionally, it was made with odds and ends from the Sunday roast, finely chopped; it would be a good use for any leftovers from the Roasted Lamb Shoulder (page 97). Grated cheddar melted on top is not traditional, of course, but with all that great Shelburne Farms cheddar around, it was a natural and delicious addition. ◇ ***Serves: 6–8***

For the caramelized onions

3 tablespoons olive oil

2 pounds onions (about 6 medium), thinly sliced crosswise into rounds

1 teaspoon coarse kosher salt

For the potato smash

3 pounds all-purpose potatoes, such as Yukon gold, scrubbed but not peeled and cut into 2-inch chunks

4 garlic cloves, smashed with the flat side of a knife

1 teaspoon coarse kosher salt plus more to taste

¼ cup (½ stick) unsalted butter, cut into 4 pieces

For the lamb filling and to finish pie

1 tablespoon olive oil

3 medium carrots, scrubbed, trimmed and finely diced (about 1½ cups)

Before You Start See A Note on Lamb (page 81) for tips on buying ground lamb. You can use a combination of ground lamb and finely chopped or ground leftover cooked lamb; just brown the cooked lamb along with the ground. And yes, it does take time to caramelize the onions, but it is absolutely worth it; they add a depth of flavor that really makes this dish special. Steaming, rather than boiling, potatoes makes for a firmer and drier mashed potato topping, although it's fine to boil them if that's easier for you. They are not as rich as many mashed potato recipes because of the lamb underneath and the cheddar on top.

1. *Make the caramelized onions (up to a week ahead):* In a large, heavy-bottomed sauté pan or skillet set over medium heat, heat the olive oil until hot. Add the onions to the pan and turn the heat down to medium-low.

2. Sprinkle the onions with the salt and cook, stirring frequently to make sure they brown evenly, for about 30–40 minutes or until they are completely golden brown and soft. You should have about 1½–2 cups of onions. Set aside.

Lamb

2 pounds ground lamb

1½ teaspoons minced fresh thyme leaves

1 teaspoon coarse kosher salt

2 tablespoons all-purpose flour

1 tablespoon tomato paste (ketchup will do in a pinch)

2 cups chicken stock, preferably low sodium

1 cup (about 3–4 ounces) grated cheddar

3. *Make the smashed potatoes (up to 24 hours ahead):* Select a large pot that can accommodate a steamer insert or heatproof colander large enough to hold your potatoes. Fill it with water up to the bottom of the steamer insert, add the potatoes and garlic cloves, and sprinkle them with the salt. Cover the pot, set it over high heat, and bring the water to a boil.

4. Reduce the heat to maintain an active simmer and steam the potatoes for 25–30 minutes until they break apart easily when poked with a fork.

5. Remove the potatoes and garlic from the steamer, pour off the hot water, and return the potatoes and garlic to the pot. Cover the potatoes with a clean dish towel and let them dry out for about 5 minutes. (Do not allow the potatoes to cool before mashing or they will get disastrously gummy.) Add the butter to the pot and use a potato masher to smash the potatoes and garlic until blended but not completely smooth. Adjust seasoning to taste. Set aside.

6. *Make the meat filling and finish the pie:* Preheat the oven to 400°F. In a large sauté pan or skillet set over medium-high heat, heat the olive oil until hot. Add the diced carrots and cook, stirring occasionally, for 5–7 minutes until softened.

7. Add the lamb, thyme, and salt, and cook, stirring occasionally, for 8–10 minutes until the meat is no longer pink. Carefully pour off all the fat and discard.

8. Sprinkle the flour over the lamb and cook for 1 minute, stirring. Then stir in the tomato paste and cook, stirring, for 2 minutes longer. Pour in the stock, along with 1 cup of the caramelized onions. Increase the heat slightly and simmer, 2–3 minutes, until the gravy thickens slightly.

9. Spread the lamb into a shallow round or oval 3-quart casserole or a 9 by 13-inch baking dish. Spread the potatoes on top. Distribute the remaining caramelized onions over the mashed potatoes, and then sprinkle the cheddar evenly on top. Bake until the top is golden and crusty, about 20 minutes.

Variation For a rich cheddar smash to serve at a different time, use the same ingredients for the smash but peel the potatoes. Follow steps 3 through 5 but mash 2–3 cups (8 ounces) of grated cheddar into the hot potatoes along with ¾ cup of warm milk or half-and-half, mixing until smooth.

> *Prepare-Ahead Tip:* In addition to the parts noted above that can be made ahead, the whole shepherd's pie can be put together up to 24 hours ahead and kept refrigerated. Start baking it at 375°F for 30 minutes to warm the pie through, and then increase to 400°F for the final 20 minutes to brown the top.

Lamb

Wild Mushrooms

- Coach Barn Sherried Mushrooms with Triple-Cream Cheese
- Chanterelles, Corn, and Goat Cheese with Tagliatelle
- Baked Mushroom and Cheese Bread Stuffing
- Mushroom and Kale Lasagna with Blue Cheese
- Scalloped Potatoes with Mushrooms and Canadian Bacon
- Mushroom and Root Vegetable Potpie
- Chicken with Roasted Garlic and Mushrooms
- Salmon with Creamed Mushrooms and Kohlrabi
- Braised Veal and Mushrooms
- Grilled Steak with Cumin-Coriander Mushrooms

*W*here there are woods and fields, there will be mushrooms. Vermont's many and varied miles of open space are the perfect habitat for morels, chanterelles, hen of the woods, and even prized white matsutakes. From spring to late fall, local foragers also gather less familiar but no less delicious varieties including the evocatively named pheasant back, pig's ear *Gomphus,* and wine-cap *Stropharia.*

Mushrooms are bewitching and challenging; people cannot quite believe that such delectable edibles grow free for the taking. Expertise, however, is critical; the price for ignorance or hubris could be death. To become a successful mushroom forager, you must be a student not only of mushrooms, but also of their environment. Most important, "you should never be afraid to say you don't know," emphasizes mushroom expert Les Hook.

At Shelburne Farms, Alec and Marshall Webb remember collecting giant puffballs from the fields when they were children. The woods continue to harbor hidden mycological treasures among the mosses, under damp leaves, and up tree trunks. As intriguing as wild mushrooms, perhaps, was the existence of a mushroom house, a greenhouse in which the Shelburne Farms gardener cultivated mushrooms at the turn of the century. The harvest would have been now-common white button mushrooms, then known as "champignons de Paris," which had come into vogue in the early nineteenth century in France and were grown in old stone quarries around that country's capital city. The practice came to the United States at the very end of the century and, as the American upper classes adopted French culinary style in their kitchens, they also followed this trend by building mushroom houses at their country estates.

Wild or cultivated, mushrooms carry a taste of the earth: from the deep woodsy morel to the pale, delicately frilled oyster. They soak up flavors but always make their own unique contribution to a dish, adding texture and depth, whether paired with an assertive blue cheese or sweet, fresh corn.

A Note on Wild Mushrooms

The world of wild mushrooms is vast, with well over twenty thousand mushroom varieties in North America and less than one third of those identified. Vermont mushroom experts Les Hook and Nova Kim sell about 150 varieties of mushrooms, which have widely varying flavors and textures. The age of a mushroom can also affect its flavor and texture significantly, as can the region from which it is gathered. We have included wild options for each recipe, as well as more commonly available cultivated mushrooms that can be substituted. There is an increasing variety of cultivated exotic mushrooms available, including oyster, hen of the woods (maitake), and even bear's head tooth. The cultivated versions are generally milder than the wild. It goes without saying, but only purchase wild mushrooms from a trusted source, and do not forage on your own without significant training or an expert guide.

The following outlines some of the main types of mushrooms that Les and Nova find during a typical Vermont season. It is meant as a guide to mushrooms you can purchase, not as a guide for mushroom foraging.

Boletus edulis is the most common in the bolete family, known as porcini in Italy and cèpes in France. They are prized for their aroma, their delicious flavor, and the texture of their solid caps and stalks. They can be sautéed, roasted, or braised.

Chanterelles and other vase-shaped mushrooms are fairly delicate with their petal-like caps and are good for a quick sauté.
- Chanterelles (*Cantharellaceae*), including trumpet (*tubaeformis*), yellow-footed (*xanthopus*), and black trumpet (*fallax*)
- Flat-topped coral (*Clavariadelphus truncatus*) is uniquely sweet and fruity.
- Pig's ear *Gomphus* (*Gomphus clavatus*)

Gilled mushrooms are the more traditional-looking capped mushrooms and can generally be cooked as you would cook button mushrooms—although they usually offer better flavor.
- Fawn (*Pluteus cervinus*)
- Honey (*Aarmillariella mellea*)
- Meadow (*Agaricus campestris*) and horse (*Agaricus arvensis*)
- Swollen or imperial cat (*Catathelasma ventricosa* or *imperialis*)
- Wine-cap *Stropharia* (*Stropharia rugosoannulata*)

- White matsutake (identified variously as *Armillaria ponderosa,*
  Tricholoma ponderoum, or *Tricholoma magnivelare*)
- Lobster mushrooms (*Hypomyces lactifluorum*) are actually a mold that
  grows on the gilled *Lactarius* and *Russula* mushrooms. They are very
  distinctive for their dark apricot color and meaty texture. They need
  quite a bit of liquid to keep from drying out while cooking and can be
  stewed or braised.
- Similarly, the snow shrimp (aborted *Entoloma*) is the parasitized form
  of the gilled *Entaloma abortivum.* It is sweet, mild, and meaty.

Morels (*Morchella*), including black, white, midget, yellow, and giant,
are hollow with distinctive honeycombed caps, which give them a unique
texture to go with their earthy, sometimes nutty flavor. They can be
baked, sautéed, or simmered in liquid. Dried morels are widely available
and usually a very good option.

Polypores and other shelf mushrooms are a diverse group.
- Chicken (*Lateiporus sulphureus,* sometimes called chicken of the woods)
  can vary greatly depending on age. Older specimens are best dried and
  ground into mushroom powder to be used like seasoned flour or bread
  crumbs or in mushroom stock. Full slices should be cut thinly; they
  are very sturdy and are best in stews and braises, where they will
  contribute a meaty, chickeny texture. The more delicate tips can be
  sautéed.
- Hen of the woods (*Grifola frondosa,* also known as maitake) are
  increasingly available cultivated and have a nice delicate texture and
  flavor that adds variety to a mix. Chunks can be roasted or smaller
  pieces sautéed.
- Pheasant back (*Polyporus squamosus,* also known as Dryad's saddle) can
  be roasted or grilled whole, or, sliced thin, they can be sautéed or
  roasted quickly.
- Oysters (*Pleurotus ostreatus*) are generally more delicate and best for
  quick cooking, but the blue pearl (*Pleurotus columbinus*) and the late-
  season green backs (*Panellus serotinus*) are meatier and should be
  cooked a little longer and more gently with a little liquid or fat.
- Umbrella polypore (*Polyporus umbellatus*) is most similar to hen of the
  woods.

Puffballs (*Clavatia gigantea* and others) are best when young, but size is no indication of age. Make sure they are white all the way through. They can be sliced or diced and sautéed, roasted, or grilled with a good amount of oil and flavoring, which they will absorb like eggplant slices, to which they are often compared. They also dry very well in slices.

Tooth fungus

- Bear's head tooth (*Hericium coralloides*) and comb tooth (*Hericium ramosum*) are soft and shaggy and unlike most of what one thinks of as mushrooms. Small pieces or slices can be sautéed or gently roasted.
- Sweet tooth (*Dentinum repandum,* also known as hedgehog) is often used where one might use chanterelles.

Preparing and Cooking Mushrooms

- Mushrooms, wild or cultivated, have a relatively short shelf life. Keep them dry and cool, wrapped loosely in a paper bag.
- Although there are a few exceptions, as a general rule, do not eat wild mushrooms raw.
- Brush mushrooms with a soft bristle brush or wipe them off with a damp cloth. The exception is morels. (See Tip below.)
- Nova and Les suggest that if you want your mushrooms to absorb flavor, cut them to break their cell structure. If you want them to retain more of their own flavor, tear them gently apart to preserve their cell structure.
- In recipes where you can substitute dry mushrooms for fresh, estimate a one-to-ten ratio, dry to fresh.
- To dry your own mushrooms, brush them and cut away any bad spots. Split morels or chanterelles in half to make sure there are no visitors. Others should be sliced as thin as possible and then either laid on a screen to ensure air circulation or dehydrated in a dehydrator. They need a temperature of about 98–100°F to dry.

Tip: *Morels should be cleaned thoroughly before use because they easily collect dirt and sand in their honeycombed caps and insects love their hollow stems. Rinse fresh or dried mushrooms several times, using a clean toothbrush to gently dislodge grit if any remains.*

Coach Barn Sherried Mushrooms with Triple-Cream Cheese

A simple and delicious way to enjoy almost any kind of mushroom and a very popular appetizer at Coach Barn receptions. As a first course, use the cheese and mushroom-topped toasts to crown a salad of spinach, arugula, or frisée. The sherried mushrooms alone make a great condiment for grilled steak or hamburger.

◇ *Serves: 4–6 as an appetizer or as part of a salad*

12 baguette slices, toasted or grilled

1 wheel of triple-cream or other soft, creamy cheese, 6–8 ounces, sliced into 12 equal wedges and brought to room temperature

2 tablespoons olive oil

¾ pound mushrooms (see Before You Start) trimmed of tough stem ends and thinly sliced

½ teaspoon coarse kosher salt plus more to taste

2 small shallots, finely minced (about 2 tablespoons)

3 cloves garlic, finely minced (about 1 tablespoon)

¾ cup dry sherry

1 tablespoon finely minced fresh thyme leaves

1 tablespoon unsalted butter

Freshly ground black pepper to taste

Before You Start Delicate wild mushrooms such as young wine-cap *Stropharia,* chanterelles, or wild oysters would be lovely, but this will also work with cultivated oyster mushrooms, and even raises the common white mushroom to new heights. We have some wonderful creamy cheeses made in Vermont in the style of triple creams, double creams, and the less rich but also good Brie and Camembert. Look for those from Champlain Valley Creamery, in the "Sweet Milk" chapter, Lazy Lady Farm of Westfield, Willow Hill Farm in Milton, and Blythedale Farm in Corinth (see Sources, page 273).

1. Lay the toasted baguette rounds on a serving platter and top with the slices of cheese.

2. Set a large sauté pan or skillet over medium-high heat and add the olive oil. When the oil is shimmering, add the mushrooms, salt, shallot, and garlic. Cook, stirring occasionally, until the mushrooms have given up their liquid and turned golden and they make a squeaking noise against the pan, 10–12 minutes.

3. Add the sherry, thyme, and butter to the pan and cook, stirring occasionally, until no liquid remains, about 5 minutes. Adjust seasoning to taste.

4. Spoon the mushrooms immediately over the toast topped with cheese, and serve.

Chanterelles, Corn, and Goat Cheese with Tagliatelle

[photograph 9]

The combination of fresh, nutty chanterelles and just-picked sweet corn with the fresh tang of goat cheese delivers summer in a bowl. ◇ ***Serves: 4***

1 pound tagliatelle

2 tablespoons olive oil

2 tablespoons unsalted butter

½ pound fresh chanterelles, whole if small or cut in half

Kernels from 4 ears fresh corn (about 2 cups) (see Tip, page 14)

½ teaspoon coarse kosher salt plus more to taste

8 slender scallions, white and pale green parts only, sliced into ½-inch lengths at an angle

1 cup (4 ounces) crumbled fresh soft goat cheese

Freshly ground black pepper to taste

Before You Start I hesitate to even offer substitute possibilities here because this is so good with the chanterelles, but wild or cultivated oysters will also work. We have many fresh local goat cheeses in Vermont, and one of the best, from Vermont Butter & Cheese in Websterville, is available nationwide. You can use thawed frozen corn in a pinch.

1. Put a large pot of salted water on to boil for the pasta. Cook the pasta according to package directions.

2. While the pasta is cooking, set a large sauté pan or skillet over medium-high heat and heat the olive oil and butter until foamy. Add the chanterelles and corn and cook, stirring occasionally, for 4–5 minutes until the mushrooms and corn are lightly colored. Add the salt and scallions and cook, stirring occasionally, for 3–4 minutes until everything is golden.

3. Before draining the pasta, scoop ½ cup of the pasta cooking liquid out of the pot and reserve it. Drain the pasta and toss it immediately into the pan with the vegetables. Sprinkle the goat cheese over the pasta along with about ¼ cup of the reserved pasta cooking liquid. Toss to coat, adding a little more liquid if desired. Adjust seasoning to taste and serve immediately.

Baked Mushroom and Cheese Bread Stuffing

This is the perfect side dish for broiled or roasted meats. It is light and savory, not heavy at all. ◇ *Serves: 4–6 as a side dish*

1½ cups half-and-half

½ ounce (a scant cup) dried chanterelle mushrooms or 5 ounces (about 1½ cups) fresh chanterelles, whole if small or cut in half

¾ pound crusty, country-style bread, trimmed of hard crusts and cut into 1-inch cubes (about 4 cups)

1 shallot, thinly sliced

2 ounces (about ½ cup) coarsely shredded, aged, lightly nutty cheese (see Before You Start)

1 teaspoon fresh thyme leaves

1 large egg

½ teaspoon coarse kosher salt

Freshly ground black pepper to taste

Before You Start   Other lightly fragranced dried or fresh exotic mushrooms, such as hen of the woods, meadow, or oyster mushrooms torn into small pieces, could be used. This is a recipe where dried mushrooms are as good as or perhaps even better than fresh. We love to make it with Tarentaise, an Alpine-style aged cow's milk cheese from Thistle Hill Farm in North Pomfret, or the nutty, aged sheep cheese from Vermont Shepherd in Putney (see Sources, page 273). A good aged Gruyère or Comté-style cheese could be substituted for the Vermont cheese.

1. Preheat the oven to 400°F. Lightly butter the bottom and sides of a 2-quart casserole dish.

2. In a medium saucepan, combine the half-and-half with the mushrooms and bring to a simmer over medium heat. Simmer for 5 minutes. (If using dried mushrooms, simmer until they are tender. This could be as little as 5 minutes or as long as 15, depending on the variety and age of the mushrooms. If you need to cook the mushrooms longer and too much of the cream reduces, add more to keep the liquid at 1½ cups.) Remove from the heat.

3. Put the bread cubes, shallot, all but 3 tablespoons of the cheese, and the thyme into a large bowl. Crack the egg into the bowl and, using your hands, break the egg and toss the mixture to combine all the ingredients well. Pour the half-and-half and mushroom mixture evenly over the bread. Add the salt and pepper to taste and stir to combine.

4. Scrape the mixture into the prepared casserole dish. Lightly butter a piece of foil and cover.

5. Bake for 15 minutes. Remove the foil and sprinkle the remaining cheese on top of the dish. Bake for another 8–10 minutes until golden. Serve immediately.

Listening to the Land
Les Hook and Nova Kim,
wildcrafters

"Sometimes you think you're never going to find another mushroom, but then you do. It's magic. I don't understand it myself."—Les Hook

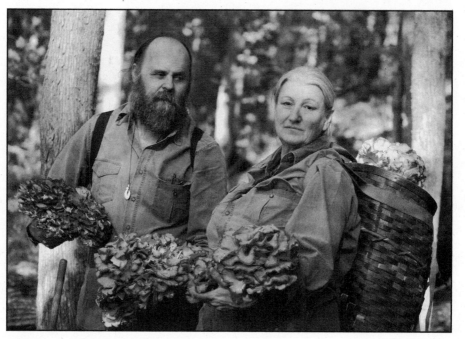

*l*es Hook and Nova Kim have a suggestion for those interested in following in their footsteps. "Take four objects," Nova says, "and hide them in the woods. Then come back and find them. People say, 'Oh, I can't do that.' But you can."

Wildcrafting (the term that Les and Nova prefer to *foraging*) "is all about scouting, being aware of your surroundings, learning to recognize when something's out of place," says Nova. "You've got to know your trees and your leaves," adds Les. "And when you come into any woods, be prepared to accept what it offers," Nova finishes.

Together, the couple has been wildcrafting mushrooms and other edible and medicinal plants for twenty-seven years, eking out a living selling (mostly to restaurants), teaching, and leading guided walks. They live largely off the grid and estimate that 85 percent of what they eat is wild. "You adjust your life to what you need," says Nova. A few years ago they tried taking on a paper route to supplement their income. "But we couldn't do it," shrugs Les. "The papers had to be there at a certain time, and we couldn't stop on the way if we saw something good."

Les has lived off the land since his childhood in rural Vermont. "My father died when I was eight, and there were nine of us. We were always eating wild food because we didn't have anything else to eat," he explains matter-of-factly. Nova, who is half Osage, believes she was drawn to wildcrafting by her tribal bloodline, but not by family example. During her Wyoming childhood, native traditions were not celebrated: "Every morning before you went to school, you were told, don't tell anyone you're native," she recalls. But Nova came to embrace her heritage and often uses an Osage phrase, *Ka-ti-na-gha,* which means, "Look for the coming of a peaceful day."

Being in the woods with Nova and Les is peaceful, although it can also be a little dizzying, as they point out edible and medicinal plants at almost every turn. "If you're walking through the woods and you smell apricot, look around for chanterelles. If you smell licorice, look up and you'll see oysters," offers Nova. "And when you see a downed beech, always look for bear's head," she says, stooping to carefully cut a shaggy specimen off a log.

Nova and Les see promise in every pile of leaves, on every tree. Gesturing to a decayed mushroom, Les says, "Even if you find something dead, come back. You'll get a bushel there next year." They are rewarded for their patience, for their persistence, and for paying attention to what the woods have to tell them. "Sometimes you think you're never going to find another mushroom, but then you do," muses Les. "It's magic. I don't understand it myself."

Nova spies a cluster of toffee-colored honey mushrooms and kneels down to pick, breaking them off gently at the root, filling the hole back in, and brushing the dirt off before putting the mushrooms into a paper bag. After harvesting a few, she observes that slugs or insects have been nibbling on them. "Somebody's eating these," she says. "We'll leave them. We have a car; they don't." She places the bag in her collecting basket and moves on. "Appreciate all the cycles of life, be mindful of animals," Nova sums up, "and never take so much that those coming behind you have nothing."

The couple is concerned for those who come behind them. Pointing out cracks in the earth, Nova shakes her head and says, "All that rain this summer, and it's still dry." They have started to record soil temperatures in an effort to understand the environmental changes they have observed, and are encouraging others to do the same. "The forest is an ever-changing landscape," she says. "Remember, for better or worse, you are an integral part of that change."

Mushroom and Kale Lasagna with Blue Cheese

Mushrooms, dark leafy greens, and rich blue cheese combine to create an earthy and hearty vegetarian lasagna. We have some lovely blue cheeses made here in Vermont, including those from Green Mountain Blue Cheese in Highgate Center and Bayley Hazen Blue from Jasper Hill Farm in Greensboro (see Sources, page 273). ◇ **Serves: 8–10**

¼ cup olive oil

3 pounds assorted mushrooms (see Before You Start), cut or torn into bite-size pieces

1 teaspoon coarse kosher salt plus more to taste

2 medium leeks, white and light green parts only, halved lengthwise, thinly sliced, and rinsed thoroughly

4 cloves garlic, cut lengthwise into thin slivers

1 pound kale, torn from tough stalks into bite-size pieces, rinsed in a colander but not dried

1 (9-ounce) box no-boil lasagna noodles (see Before You Start)

¼ cup (½ stick) unsalted butter

¼ cup all-purpose flour

4 cups milk, not skim

2 cups (about 8 ounces) crumbled blue cheese

Freshly ground black pepper to taste

½ cup (about 2–3 ounces) freshly grated Parmesan

Before You Start   Pretty much any mushroom that will sauté well will work in this recipe, and a mix of mushrooms is especially good here, even some dry reconstituted tossed in with the fresh after they've been sautéed. (Nova and Les recommend thinly sliced, dried puffballs.) I like the ease of no-boil lasagna noodles, although I have borrowed a tip from the thorough test kitchen at *Cook's Illustrated* and soak them for a little while to soften them up before I use them. Quality of the no-boil kind varies; I have always had great success with Barilla brand. If you prefer regular noodles, by all means go ahead and boil away.

1. Preheat the oven to 400°F. Lightly oil a 9 by 13-inch baking dish.

2. In a large sauté pan or skillet, heat 3 tablespoons of the olive oil over medium-high heat. Add the mushrooms, starting with the most sturdy varieties, sprinkling them with ½ teaspoon of the salt. Give them about 5 minutes' head start, then add the more delicate varieties. Cook, stirring occasionally, until the mushrooms have given up their liquid and turned golden and they make a squeaking noise against the pan, up to an additional 12–15 minutes. Remove the mushrooms from the pan to a bowl and set aside.

3. Put the same large pan back over medium-high heat with the remaining tablespoon of olive oil. Add the leeks and slivered garlic to the pan and sauté until soft, 2–3 minutes. Add the kale to the pan with the remaining ½ teaspoon salt and turn it with tongs to wilt it evenly, cooking for 3–4 minutes. (If the pan gets too dry, add a little water.) Cover the pan, reduce the heat to medium-low, and cook for an additional 5–7 minutes until the kale is tender. Remove the cover and set aside.

4. Put the lasagna noodles in a large colander and set the colander in a large bowl. Fill the bowl with hot tap water and soak the lasagna noodles for about 10 minutes while you make the sauce.

5. In a medium saucepan set over medium-high heat, melt the butter until foamy. Whisk in the flour and cook, 1–2 minutes, until golden. Gradually whisk in the milk and bring to a simmer. When the sauce reaches a simmer, whisk briskly until the sauce thickens slightly, about 2–3 minutes. Take the pot off the heat and whisk in 1¾ cups of the crumbled blue cheese. Add a few grinds of black pepper to taste.

6. Start building the lasagna in the prepared pan by lightly coating the bottom with 1 cup of the blue cheese sauce. Lay four drained noodles on top of the sauce, followed by ⅓ of the sautéed mushrooms, ⅓ of the sautéed kale, and 2 tablespoons of the grated Parmesan. Repeat twice. Finish with the last four lasagna noodles and the remaining sauce. Spread the sauce to cover the noodles and sprinkle the remaining Parmesan and blue cheese over the top.

7. Cover the lasagna with foil and bake for 30 minutes. Remove the foil carefully and bake for an additional 20 minutes until golden and bubbling. Let stand for 5 minutes before serving.

> **Prepare-Ahead Tip:** *The whole lasagna can be prepared a day ahead and refrigerated unbaked. Add an extra 20 minutes to the baking time under the foil.*

Scalloped Potatoes with Mushrooms and Canadian Bacon

An old New England wintertime favorite, speckled with the deep earthiness of mushrooms. This version was modeled after one in Jane Grigson's classic book, The Mushroom Feast, *which intrigued me because she dispenses with the step of sautéeing the mushrooms—and it works.* ◇ ***Serves: 4 as a main dish, 6–8 as a side dish***

1½ pounds starchy potatoes such as Russet, peeled and sliced very thin, about ⅛ inch thick

1 clove garlic, finely chopped

½ teaspoon coarse kosher salt

½ pound mixed mushrooms (see Before You Start), thinly sliced

Freshly ground black pepper to taste

6 ounces Canadian bacon slices

¾ cup heavy cream

¾ cup half-and-half

¾ cup (about 3 ounces) grated cheddar or aged Colby-style cheese

Before You Start   This recipe can accommodate a variety of mushrooms. On the wild side, try hen of the woods, honey mushrooms, or wine-cap *Stropharia*. Cremini or white button with some cultivated oysters for variation will work too. Make sure to use starchy potatoes; the waxy kind won't work at all. We like to make this with Shelburne Farms cheddar, particularly the two-year, but we also like to top it with another Vermont farmstead cheese, Orb Weaver's farmhouse-aged Colby-style cheese (see Sources, page 273) with its hint of grass and beautiful melting texture.

1. Preheat the oven to 375°F. Generously butter a 1½–2 quart shallow casserole dish.

2. Arrange half of the potatoes overlapping to form one layer in the bottom of the prepared dish. Sprinkle with the garlic and season with ¼ teaspoon of salt. Spread the mushrooms evenly over the potatoes and season with a few grinds of pepper to taste. Arrange the Canadian bacon in one layer over the mushrooms and finish with the remaining potatoes overlapping to form a final layer.

3. In a small bowl, whisk together the heavy cream and half-and-half and pour the liquid carefully and evenly over the potatoes. The liquid will not come to the top of the potatoes. Sprinkle with the remaining ¼ teaspoon of salt, and then spread the cheese evenly over the top. (If your casserole dish is filled all the way to the top, put a cookie sheet on the oven shelf below to catch any bubbling overflow.)

4. Bake in the oven for 65–75 minutes until bubbly and deep golden brown and a fork easily pierces a potato slice. Let sit for 5–10 minutes before serving.

Mushroom and Root Vegetable Potpie

A satisfying stew of meaty mushrooms and sweet, roasted root vegetables. The Cheddar and Herb Biscuits are a great topper and make this our homage to the chicken pies served at church suppers all over Vermont, which are always finished with fluffy biscuits baked on top. ◇ *Serves: 8–10*

Cheddar and Herb Biscuits (page 24), made with fresh thyme and cut into twelve 2-inch rounds

3 pounds assorted root vegetables, such as carrots, turnips, rutabagas, beets, parsnips, and sweet potatoes, peeled and cut into 1-inch cubes

3 tablespoons olive oil

1 tablespoon coarsely chopped fresh thyme leaves

1½ teaspoons coarse kosher salt plus more to taste

Freshly ground black pepper to taste

6 tablespoons unsalted butter

3 medium leeks, white and light green parts only, halved lengthwise, thinly sliced, and rinsed thoroughly

2 pounds mixed mushrooms, quartered or torn into bite-size pieces (see Before You Start)

3 tablespoons all-purpose flour

4 cups mushroom stock or vegetable stock (see Before You Start)

Before You Start   This dish can take a wide variety of mushrooms and, in fact, works best with a variety of those on the sturdy side, such as cultivated cremini and white buttons as well as wild pheasant back, thin slices of chicken mushrooms, and a mixture of gilled mushrooms. If you cannot find prepackaged mushroom stock—which is available in some supermarkets and natural foods stores either in concentrate or in cartons—warm the vegetable stock and soak one ounce of your choice of dried mushrooms in it for about 20 minutes. Finely mince the reconstituted dried mushrooms and add them to the sautéed mushroom-leek mixture with the stock. The filling must be hot when you put the biscuits on it, or the biscuit bottoms will get gummy.

1. Make the Cheddar and Herb Biscuits, but do not brush them with the buttermilk yet. Cover the biscuits with a damp towel and refrigerate.

2. Preheat the oven to 400°F. Toss together the root vegetables in a 9 by 13-inch baking dish with 2 tablespoons of the olive oil, the thyme, 1 teaspoon of the salt, and pepper to taste. Roast for 40–45 minutes, or until a fork easily pierces a piece of each vegetable. (Some may be softer than others.) Take the vegetables out of the oven and increase the heat to 425°F.

3. While the root vegetables are roasting, set a large sauté pan or skillet over medium-high heat and melt 1 tablespoon of the butter until foamy. Add the leeks and cook, stirring occasionally, until softened, about 3–4 minutes.

4. Add the mushrooms to the pan along with the remaining tablespoon of olive oil, starting with the most sturdy varieties and sprinkling them with the remaining ½ teaspoon of salt. Give them about a 5-minute head start, and then add more delicate varieties. Cook, stirring occasionally, until the mushrooms have given up their liquid and turned golden and they make a squeaking noise against the pan, up to an additional 10–12 minutes.

5. Reduce the heat to medium and add the remaining 5 tablespoons of butter to the pan. When the butter has melted, stir in the flour and cook for 1–2 minutes until the flour is golden. Stir in the mushroom stock and bring to a simmer. Cook, stirring, for 4–5 minutes, until the gravy thickens. Adjust seasoning to taste.

6. Pour the mushroom gravy over the roasted root vegetables in the baking dish and stir to combine. Arrange the prepared biscuits on top of the hot filling. Brush the biscuits with buttermilk. Bake for 15–20 minutes until the biscuits are golden brown and the filling is bubbly.

> **Prepare-Ahead Tip:** You can prepare the filling up to 24 hours ahead and keep it in the refrigerator. Warm the filling, covered with foil, in a 425°F oven for 30 minutes before adding the biscuits.

Chicken with Roasted Garlic and Mushrooms

Roasted mushrooms are not beautiful, but they develop a deep, concentrated flavor that more than makes up for their wrinkles. The mushroom stuffing adds a second layer of foresty flavor to this dish and also keeps the chicken breast nice and moist. ◇ *Serves: 4*

4 slices thick-cut bacon (about ¼ pound)

¾ pound mixed mushrooms and tender stems, coarsely chopped, plus ½ pound sturdy mushrooms for roasting around chicken, halved if small or cut into ½-inch pieces (see Before You Start)

3 small shallots, minced (about 3 tablespoons)

1 tablespoon minced fresh thyme leaves plus 1 tablespoon whole fresh thyme leaves

Roasted garlic squeezed from the cloves of 1 large head of garlic (see Tip, page 123)

4 bone-in, skin-on chicken breast halves (about ¾ pound each)

1½ teaspoons coarse kosher salt

Freshly ground black pepper to taste

1 teaspoon freshly squeezed lemon juice

Before You Start This stuffing works well with the most humble of mushrooms and is a good way to use up leftover mushroom stems. For the mushrooms to roast around the chicken, halved cremini or thick chunks of portobellos (which are simply larger creminis) will do fine, or look for cultivated or wild hen of the woods, chicken mushrooms, or pheasant backs. For an extra treat, fresh *Boletus edulis* or morels would take this dish to another level altogether. For easiest stuffing, try to find chicken breasts with skin that is as intact as possible.

1. In a medium skillet or sauté pan set over medium-high heat, cook the bacon until crisp. Set it aside on paper towel to drain and discard all but 2 tablespoons of the bacon fat.

2. Put the pan with the bacon fat back over medium-high heat and add the coarsely chopped mushrooms. Cook, stirring occasionally, until the mushrooms have given up their liquid and turned golden and they make a squeaking noise against the pan, 8–10 minutes. Add the shallots and minced thyme leaves and continue to cook for 3–4 minutes until the shallots are softened.

3. Preheat the oven to 425°F. Put the mushroom mixture into a food processor with the garlic and process for about 10 seconds just until combined and finely minced. Crumble the bacon and add it to the food processor, pulsing 3–4 times just to coarsely chop the bacon and distribute it throughout the stuffing.

4. Tuck about ⅓ cup of the stuffing under the skin of each chicken breast. Season the skin with 1 teaspoon of the salt and pepper to taste and place the breasts skin up in a large baking or roasting pan surrounded by the remaining ½ pound of mushrooms. Sprinkle the mushrooms with the whole thyme leaves, the remaining tablespoon of olive oil, and the remaining ½ teaspoon of salt.

5. Roast the chicken and mushrooms for 35–40 minutes until the chicken is cooked through or the meat registers 165°F on an instant-read thermometer. Squeeze the lemon juice over the chicken right before serving.

> **Tip:** To roast whole garlic bulbs, slice off the top of the bulb to expose the clove interiors, wrap the bulb in foil with a splash of olive oil and a sprinkle of coarse kosher salt, and roast at 375°F for about 40 minutes until the cloves are very soft and you can easily squeeze them out of their skins. A large garlic bulb should yield about 3–4 tablespoons of roasted garlic.
>
> **Prepare-Ahead Tip:** The stuffing can be made ahead and kept refrigerated for two or three days.

Wild Mushrooms

Salmon with Creamed Mushrooms and Kohlrabi

Creamed mushrooms are so good, and they work beautifully with this pan-poached salmon. We love the contrast between the soft, earthy mushrooms, the moist salmon, and the firm, nutty nuggets of kohlrabi, which is a sadly neglected vegetable. ◇ *Serves: 4*

2 skinned, center-cut salmon fillets (1½–2 pounds total), preferably wild, any visible pin bones removed with tweezers

1½ teaspoons coarse kosher salt plus more to taste

1 tablespoon olive oil

2 medium shallots, thinly sliced

2 medium kohlrabies (about ¾ pound), peeled and cut into ½-inch cubes

8 ounces delicate mushrooms (see Before You Start), trimmed of any tough stems and torn into bite-size pieces

1 cup dry white wine

1 cup heavy cream

Freshly ground black pepper to taste

Before You Start   Use a fairly delicate mushroom here. Cultivated or wild oysters will do nicely, as will small wild honey mushrooms or sweet tooth (also known as hedgehog), which will add a light, sweet note to the dish. If you cannot find kohlrabi, this dish works well with sunchokes. They are the cultivated relative of Jerusalem artichokes, which can be dug from the wild in Vermont.

1. Pat the salmon dry and season both sides with 1 teaspoon of the salt.

2. In a large sauté pan or skillet set over medium-high heat, heat the olive oil until hot. Add the shallot and sauté until softened, 3–4 minutes. Add the kohlrabi cubes and cook, stirring occasionally, until the cubes start to color, about 7–9 minutes.

3. Add the mushrooms to the pan with the remaining ½ teaspoon salt and cook, continuing to stir occasionally, until the mushrooms have given up their liquid and started to color, another 7–9 minutes. Pour the white wine into the pan and simmer for 5 minutes.

4. Reduce the heat to medium-low. Lay the salmon fillets on top of the kohlrabies and mushrooms and pour the cream over the fish. Cover and simmer for 10–15 minutes, until the salmon is just cooked through. Adjust seasoning to taste and serve immediately.

From the Archives: Creamed mushrooms have long been a classic. Lila Webb's book-plated copy of *The Waldorf-Astoria Cookbook,* published in 1896, includes boiled mushrooms in cream, mushrooms stewed in cream, and mushrooms under glass with cream. There were, however, apparently not enough recipes to deal with the abundant supply of mushrooms grown at Shelburne Farms. In December 1908, Lila Webb wrote from New York, "The amount of mushrooms sent down for the last three weeks has been ludicrous were it not also vexatious . . . if we ate nothing but mushrooms steadily, we could not begin to consume them."

Braised Veal and Mushrooms

A warming but light-tasting stew perfect for late spring or fall, when mushrooms and spinach are among the first—or the last—fresh foods to come from the earth. ◇ *Serves: 4–6*

¼ cup all-purpose flour

1½ teaspoons coarse kosher salt plus more to taste

Freshly ground black pepper to taste

1½ pounds veal stew meat, preferably from the shoulder, cut into 1-inch chunks

¼ cup olive oil

8 ounces mushrooms (see Before You Start), trimmed and torn or cut into bite-size pieces

1 small onion, cut into ½-inch chunks

2 cloves garlic, sliced

1 cup dry white wine

2 cups chicken stock, preferably low sodium

1 tablespoon Dijon mustard

1 tablespoon chopped fresh thyme leaves

8 ounces spinach leaves, tough stems removed

Before You Start   For the mushrooms, cremini will work, or go for larger wild honeys or other gilled varieties. Fresh *Boletus edulis* would also be amazing here. You can also make the stew with boneless, skinless chicken thighs, which will take about half the time in the oven.

1. Preheat the oven to 325°F. Pour the flour into a shallow, rimmed plate or pie pan and whisk in 1 teaspoon of the salt and a few grinds of pepper. Pat the veal dry and dredge it lightly in the flour mixture.

2. In a large ovenproof sauté pan or skillet, heat 2 tablespoons of the olive oil over medium-high heat. When the oil is shimmering, add the mushrooms and the remaining ½ teaspoon of salt. Cook, stirring occasionally, for 4–5 minutes. Add the onion and garlic to the pan and cook until they are soft and just colored and the mushrooms are golden brown, another 7–9 minutes. Remove the mushrooms, onions, and garlic to a bowl and set aside.

3. Put the same large pan back over medium-high heat with the remaining 2 tablespoons of olive oil. When the oil is hot, brown the veal, in batches if necessary so as not to crowd. Cook without moving the meat until a nice golden brown crust develops, 2–3 minutes on each side.

4. Add the wine and deglaze the pan, stirring to scrape up any brown bits. Simmer for 2–3 minutes. Return the mushrooms, onions, and garlic back to the pan with any accumulated juices. Add the chicken stock and bring to a simmer. Stir in the mustard and thyme.

5. Cover the pan with a lid and braise for about 90 minutes, until the veal is very tender. Remove the pan from the oven and stir in the spinach leaves. Cover the pot and let it sit for 5 minutes until the spinach is wilted. Adjust seasoning to taste and serve.

Prepare-Ahead Tip: Like almost every braise, this is even better if you make it ahead. Prepare it without the spinach, chill it, and reheat it, covered, on low heat. Stir the spinach in right before serving.

Grilled Steak with Cumin-Coriander Mushrooms

[photograph 10]

This is a quick, easy recipe that is most rewarding when made with a variety of mushrooms. British food writer Elizabeth David inspired the coriander seasoning, for which mushrooms have a wonderful affinity. Serve the steak and mushrooms on a bed of arugula or baby spinach leaves. ◇ **Serves: 4**

2 tablespoons whole coriander seeds

1 tablespoon whole cumin seeds

Freshly ground black pepper to taste

1 tablespoon minced garlic (about 3 cloves)

2 skirt steaks, about 1½–2 pounds total

1½ teaspoons coarse kosher salt plus more to taste

3 tablespoons olive oil plus more as needed

¾ pound mixed mushrooms (see Before You Start)

2 teaspoons freshly squeezed lemon juice

Parsley Sauce (page 177) if desired

Before You Start   You can use almost any mix of wild or exotic cultivated mushrooms as long as they are not too delicate. Larger pieces of oyster mushrooms, honeys, pig's ear *Gomphus,* and slices of hen of the woods work well. Skirt steak is a very reasonably priced cut of steak that has recently become more widely available in supermarkets thanks to the fact that it is used for fajitas. It is flavorful, lean, and very thin. It cooks in a flash and becomes tough if overcooked, so do not even think about taking it past medium. As Rick says, "This is a meat-eater's meat." Flank steak can be used instead, but since it's thicker, it will take a little longer to cook.

1. Prepare a gas or charcoal grill to cook over medium-high heat. Alternatively, place a large broiler-proof skillet, preferably cast iron, on the oven rack in the second-highest position, about 4–5 inches from the heating element. Preheat the broiler on its highest setting for at least 15 minutes.

2. With a mortar and pestle or a spice grinder, crush the coriander and cumin seeds together. Add about 10 grinds of pepper to the mixture and stir in the minced garlic. Take 2 teaspoons of the rub and set it aside.

3. Lay the skirt steaks on a platter and slice them into pieces that will be manageable on the grill. (Generally, each steak will do best cut into two long pieces of about 8–12 inches.) Sprinkle the steaks well with 1 teaspoon of the salt, and then apply the rub evenly on both sides of the steaks. Drizzle them evenly with 1 tablespoon of the olive oil and rub it in with your fingers. Set aside.

4. Tear the mushrooms into bite-size pieces or slice caps into ¼-inch slices, leaving smaller ones whole.

5. In a large skillet or sauté pan, heat the remaining 2 tablespoons of olive oil over medium-high heat for about 2 minutes. Add the mushrooms to the pan, along with the remaining ½ teaspoon salt and reserved 2 teaspoons of the rub. Cook, stirring occasionally, until the mushrooms have given up their liquid and turned golden and they make a squeaking noise against the pan, 10–12 minutes. Stir in the lemon juice and cover the pot to keep the mushrooms warm while grilling the steak.

6. Grill or broil the steak for 4–5 minutes per side. Let the steak rest for 10 minutes, loosely covered with foil to keep it warm. Slice the steak very thinly across the grain and serve it topped with the mushrooms and Parsley Sauce (page 177) if desired.

Game
and
Fish

- Braised Rabbit with Artichokes, Capers, and Lemon
- Rabbit, Turnip, and Bacon Stew
- Duck Breast with Tart Apples and Hard Cider
- Roast Duck Legs with Sour Cherry Sauce
- Sage and Garlic Pan-Roasted Quail
- Juniper and Maple Venison Steaks
- Venison Medallions with Cranberry Sauce
- Venison Chili
- Cornmeal Fried Trout with Bacon and Sage
- Whole Roast Trout with Ramps and Herbs

*i*t is not unusual to drive through the North Gate of Shelburne Farms and look to your left across the pasture to see the silhouette of a graceful white-tailed deer. For most visitors, the deer is a lovely sight, a reminder that wild animals still roam free, even as open land diminishes around the region. Marshall Webb, great-grandson of Lila and Seward Webb and woodlands manager for the property, has a more complicated reaction.

Over the last thirty years, development around Shelburne Farms has driven more deer to seek refuge on the Farm. At the same time, the transformation of the Farm into a public, education-oriented destination and the prohibition of firearms on Shelburne Point have precluded the hunting that previously kept the herd in check. Browsing deer started making a significant dent in new forest growth across the property during the 1980s, and a subsequent deer count by the state wildlife department confirmed that there were about double the number of deer per square mile considered healthy for a diverse northern forest.

In order to maintain vital and productive woodlands, as well as protect smaller animals like rabbits, grouse, and songbirds, something had to be done about the spiraling deer population. It was a tough situation, Marshall reflects, with "much to teach us about ecosystem integrity, the delicate dance between humans and nature, and the definition of stewardship." After considering various options, the

Farm's trustees decided to open the property to a carefully screened group of hunters for the three-week bow hunting season. "Hunting best replicates the predator-prey relationship deer have evolved with," Vermont state wildlife biologist John Buck said at the time. "It closely associates people with the value of the land and with deer as a traditional food source." Bow hunting, by its nature, is quiet, and it requires hunters to be very close to their target, ensuring the greatest possible safety for visitors to the Farm.

Bow hunting also harkens back to the earliest form of deer hunting in Vermont, as practiced by the indigenous Abenaki, who depended on wildlife including the once-abundant Atlantic salmon that returned each year to spawn before dams and polluted waterways put them on the endangered species list. Early settlers followed the Abenaki's example, and Vermont still has an active community of fishermen and hunters who hunt everything from quail to cottontail rabbits to black bears. Seward Webb was an avid hunter, as one can tell from the impressive trophies hung on the walls of the Game Room at the Inn. However, most of his large game hunting was done in places other than Vermont, on trips out West or at the family's forty-thousand-acre private hunting preserve in the Adirondacks. At Shelburne Farms, the focus was on small game, including farm-raised pheasant, quail, grouse, rabbit, and duck.

In Vermont, what is killed is almost always eaten, and community game suppers even offer tastes of raccoon, muskrat, and squirrel. Long weekends away at deer camp are legendary, and a young hunter's first buck is cause for major celebration—and lots of venison stew or chili. During the winter, small huts sprout up along the frozen edges of Lake Champlain from which hardy souls fish through the ice for perch, smelt, trout, and hatchery-bred salmon. In mid-April, anglers start fly-fishing for trout in rivers and streams, and in October, camouflaged boats slowly purr through lakes in search of duck. In addition to wild-caught game, Vermont produces farmed rabbit, quail, pheasant, and venison—even bison, although clearly those animals are not of native origin.

A Note on Game

Unless you are a hunter yourself or know someone who is, you will not be cooking true wild game, since it cannot be sold at retail in the United States. In general, farm-raised game meats such as venison, quail, and rabbit will be a little less lean than their wild counterparts, who move more and eat less. Either way, the key thing to understand about wild or farm-raised game is that—with the exception of farm-raised duck—it tends to be very lean, and when you're using dry heat like grilling or panfrying you want to be very careful not to overcook it or you'll be eating shoe leather.

Braised Rabbit with Artichokes, Capers, and Lemon

[photograph 11]

Rabbit season in Vermont runs from the end of September to early March, but rabbits are most often hunted in snowy conditions because they are easier to spot. By March, this warm braise with lighter flavors and lemony hints of spring makes for a nice supper. ◇ **Serves: 4**

¼ cup all-purpose flour

1 teaspoon coarse kosher salt plus more to taste

Freshly ground black pepper to taste

1 rabbit, about 3 pounds, cut into 6 pieces: 4 legs and 2 loin pieces

¼ cup plus 2 tablespoons olive oil

3–4 large shallots, halved and thinly sliced crosswise (about ½ cup)

1 (9-ounce) package frozen artichoke hearts, thawed and halved if they come whole

10 large caperberries with stems, sliced in half, or 2 tablespoons small capers, drained and rinsed

1 whole lemon, washed well, cut in half lengthwise and then into thin half-moons

2 tablespoons chopped fresh thyme leaves

1 cup dry white wine

1 cup chicken stock, preferably low sodium

Before You Start   Rabbits have a fairly high proportion of bone to meat; so if you are feeding especially hungry people, you may want to add another half a rabbit to the pot. For Vermont-raised farmed rabbit, see Sources (page 273). Skinless, bone-in chicken thighs make a good substitute for rabbit. Do not use jarred, marinated artichoke hearts; if you can't find frozen ones, look for the kind that come canned in water. Searching out large Spanish caperberries is well worth it.

1. Preheat the oven to 350°F. Pour the flour into a shallow, rimmed plate or pie pan and whisk in the salt and a few grinds of pepper. Pat the rabbit dry and dredge the pieces lightly in the flour mixture.

2. In a large ovenproof sauté pan or skillet, heat ¼ cup of the olive oil over medium-high heat until hot. Add the rabbit pieces and sear until golden brown, about 5 minutes per side. Remove the browned rabbit to a plate.

3. Add the remaining 2 tablespoons of olive oil to the pan and lower the heat to medium. Add the sliced shallots and cook, stirring occasionally, until golden, 3–4 minutes. Add the artichoke hearts, caperberries, lemon slices, thyme leaves, white wine, and chicken stock. Simmer for 5 minutes to reduce.

4. Return the rabbit legs—but not the loin pieces—to the pan. Place the pan in the oven and cook, covered, for 15 minutes. Add the loin pieces back to the pan, spoon cooking liquid over the meat, and cook, uncovered, for 20 minutes more until the rabbit is tender when pierced with a fork.

5. Adjust seasoning to taste and serve over mashed potatoes or with crusty bread to sop up the sauce.

> **Prepare-Ahead Tip:** *This recipe can be made entirely ahead and kept in the refrigerator for up to a day to be reheated, covered, in a 350°F oven for about 30 minutes.*

Rabbit, Turnip, and Bacon Stew

This warming mid-winter stew takes advantage of root-cellar vegetables like turnips, which were kept in every Vermont root cellar and would have been on hand during rabbit season. Long cooking mellows the bite of the turnip, although you could substitute milder rutabaga, cubed celery root, or even potatoes if you prefer. ◇ *Serves: 4*

4 ounces slab bacon, cut into ¼-inch dice, or about 4 slices thick-cut bacon, cut into ½-inch strips

1 pound turnips (about 2–3 medium), peeled and cut into ½-inch cubes

12 pearl onions, peeled, root end trimmed but left intact, halved

2 tablespoons olive oil

¼ cup all-purpose flour

1 teaspoon coarse kosher salt plus more to taste

Freshly ground black pepper to taste

1 rabbit, about 3 pounds, cut into 6 pieces: 4 legs and 2 loin pieces

12 large fresh sage leaves

1 cup dry white wine

3 cups chicken stock, preferably low sodium

2 tablespoons honey

Before You Start   See Braised Rabbit with Artichokes, Capers, and Lemon (page 136) for information on feeding a hungry crowd or substituting chicken for rabbit. Although it may be tempting to use peeled, frozen baby onions, don't do it; they will turn into mush.

1. Set a large sauté pan or skillet over medium-high heat. Add the bacon to the pan and cook until almost crisp. Pour off all but 1 tablespoon of the bacon fat and discard. Put the pan with the bacon back over the heat. Add the turnips and onions to the pan and cook, stirring occasionally, until the vegetables are lightly colored, 5–7 minutes. Remove the bacon and vegetables to a plate.

2. Keep the pan over medium-high heat and add the oil. Pour the flour into a shallow rimmed plate or pie pan and whisk in 1 teaspoon of the salt and a few grinds of pepper. Pat the rabbit dry and dredge the pieces lightly in the flour mixture. Add the rabbit pieces to the hot oil and sear until golden brown, about 5 minutes per side. Remove the browned rabbit to the plate with the bacon and vegetables.

3. Add the sage leaves to the pan and cook just until crisp, about 1 minute. Add the wine and deglaze the pan, stirring to scrape up any brown bits. Simmer for 2–3 minutes. Return the rabbit, bacon, and vegetables with any accumulated juices to the pan, along with the chicken stock. Bring to a simmer and cover the pan with the lid slightly ajar.

4. Reduce the heat to medium-low and simmer for about 45 minutes, or until the rabbit and turnips are both very tender. (You should be able to put a sharp knife into the rabbit and pull it out easily, but the meat will not fall off the bone.)

5. Remove the rabbit and vegetables to a serving bowl and cover them loosely with foil. Increase the heat to medium-high and simmer the cooking liquid for 7–10 minutes to reduce it by about half. Stir in the honey. Return the rabbit, vegetables, and bacon to the pan to warm through. Adjust seasoning to taste and serve.

> **Prepare-Ahead Tip:** *This stew can be made ahead and kept in the refrigerator for up to a day to be reheated, covered, in a 350°F oven for about 30 minutes.*

Duck Breast with Tart Apples and Hard Cider

Apple season is winding down in Vermont as duck season starts in October, and a good tart apple recently picked from the tree makes a perfect foil for the rich meat. The sweet acidity of Vermont-made hard cider in the sauce rounds it all out.

◇ *Serves: 4–6*

4 boneless, skin-on duck breasts, 8 ounces each

2 teaspoons coarse kosher salt plus more to taste

Freshly ground black pepper to taste

1 tablespoon olive oil

1 large tart apple, such as Rhode Island Greening or Granny Smith

2 medium shallots, thinly sliced

2 teaspoons finely chopped fresh rosemary leaves

1 cup hard cider (see Before You Start)

2 teaspoons honey

1 teaspoon cider vinegar

Before You Start   Hard cider varies in alcohol percentage and can be found in the beer or sparkling wine sections of some stores. See Sources (page 273) for some Vermont brands. If you cannot find hard cider, use a cup of apple cider or natural apple juice and add a little more cider vinegar at the end to balance the sweetness. If you don't have a roasting rack or other rack that fits into your sauté pan, roll a long piece of foil into a tube and form it into a large W shape to serve as an impromptu rack. We must thank Florence Fabricant for the slow-roasting method that popped up in one of her *New York Times* columns just as we were finalizing this recipe. Although you won't use the rendered duck fat in this recipe, you may want to save it for a rainy day and an indulgent snack of duck fat–roasted potatoes.

1. Preheat the oven to 200°F. With a sharp knife, score the skin and fat on each duck breast in a crisscross pattern, but do not cut into the flesh. Season the duck well on both sides with 1½ teaspoons of the salt and a few grinds of pepper.

2. Select a large ovenproof sauté pan or skillet in which you can fit a shallow roasting rack to hold the duck off the pan bottom—or see Before You Start above. Set the pan over medium-high heat, add the olive oil, and heat 2–3 minutes until hot. Add the duck, skin side down, and sear, without moving, for about 4–5 minutes until deep golden brown. If the fat gets too deep while you're searing, carefully pour it off.

3. Transfer the duck to a plate and pour off all the fat from the pan. Place the roasting rack in the pan. Set the duck on the rack, skin side up, and put it in the oven. Roast for 45–50 minutes until the duck is medium-rare or registers 165°F on an instant-read thermometer. Set the duck on a plate to rest while you make the sauce.

4. While the duck is roasting, core but do not peel the apple and slice it into half-moons ⅛-inch thick. Pour off all but 1 tablespoon of fat from the pan and place the pan over medium heat. Add the apples and cook, turning occasionally, until they are golden, about 3–4 minutes. Add the shallots and rosemary and cook, stirring, for 1–2 minutes until the shallots soften. Add the hard cider and increase the heat to reach a simmer. Simmer for 4–5 minutes. Stir in the honey, cider vinegar, and remaining ½ teaspoon of salt. Simmer for another minute. Adjust seasoning to taste.

5. Slice the duck thinly crosswise and serve topped with the apples and sauce.

Roast Duck Legs with Sour Cherry Sauce

[photograph 1 2]

A few apple orchards in Vermont grow sour cherries, and the fruit has such devoted fans that the trees are often picked clean within days of its July ripening. The tart edge of sour cherries is a natural fit for duck, and this dish makes an elegant and colorful company meal served with Honey-Glazed Carrots and Turnips (page 197) and braised kale or chard splashed with a touch of sherry vinegar (follow the kale preparation method in the Mushroom and Kale Lasagna with Blue Cheese recipe on page 116). ◇ **Serves: 4**

2 medium oranges, washed well

2 teaspoons whole fennel seeds

1 teaspoon coarse kosher salt plus more to taste

1 teaspoon sugar

2 teaspoons minced garlic

4 large duck legs, about 3½–4 pounds total

1 cup pitted fresh, thawed frozen, or canned sour cherries or ¾ cup unsweetened dried sour cherries (see Before You Start)

½ cup orange liqueur, such as Grand Marnier

1 tablespoon olive oil

4 medium shallots, thinly sliced

½ cup chicken stock, preferably low sodium

Freshly ground black pepper to taste

Before You Start   The duck legs need a minimum cure of two hours and will be most delicious and crisp if you have time to cure them overnight. Leaving them uncovered in the refrigerator dries out the skin for a much crisper result—and who doesn't appreciate that? People are most familiar with duck legs prepared confit-style, submerged in fat and cooked very slowly. This recipe, while also rich, will yield a different and slightly drier texture. If you miss the short window for fresh sour cherries, look for frozen or canned Montmorency cherries in the supermarket. Dried cherries also work, but be sure to buy the unsweetened kind, found most easily at natural foods markets.

1. Preferably the night before, and at least 2 hours before cooking, prepare the rub. Zest both oranges to yield 4 teaspoons of finely grated orange zest, making sure to avoid the bitter white pith. Wrap the zested oranges tightly in plastic wrap to prevent them from drying out and put them and 2 teaspoons of the zest in the refrigerator.

2. Finely grind the fennel seeds with the salt and sugar in a mortar and pestle or spice grinder, and then grind in the garlic and the 2 remaining teaspoons of the orange zest. Rub the mixture all over the duck legs and cure them overnight in the refrigerator, uncovered.

3. Preheat the oven to 325°F. Squeeze ½ cup of juice from the previously zested oranges into a small bowl and set aside or, if using dried cherries, stir in the orange liqueur, add the dried cherries, and set aside.

4. Set the cured duck legs on a rack in a shallow roasting pan, skin side up, and roast until the skin is crisp and dark golden brown and the meat is very tender, 2¼–2½ hours, depending on the size of the legs. (Turn a leg over and stick a sharp knife in the flesh. If the flesh still grabs the knife, the meat has not reached optimal tenderness.) About halfway through cooking, carefully pour off the fat from the roasting pan and discard or keep for another use.

5. When the duck has about 15 minutes to go, make the sauce. In a medium sauté pan, heat the olive oil over medium heat. Add the shallots and cook, stirring, for about 4–5 minutes, until they start to turn golden.

6. Add the cherries with the orange juice and orange liqueur. Stir in the remaining 2 teaspoons of orange zest and the chicken stock. Increase the heat and simmer until reduced by half, about 8–10 minutes. Adjust seasoning and serve the duck legs with the sauce.

Sage and Garlic Pan-Roasted Quail

An appetizer version of this quail is very popular at the Inn, where Rick serves it over arugula with warm sherry vinaigrette. ◇ **Serves: 4 as a main course, 8 as an appetizer**

8 semi-boneless quail, about 2 pounds total, or 2 Cornish game hens, about 1 pound each (see Tip, page 145)

20 large fresh sage leaves

4 garlic cloves, smashed with the flat side of a large knife

2 teaspoons coarse kosher salt plus more to taste

Freshly ground black pepper to taste

¼ cup olive oil

2 tablespoons unsalted butter

1 tablespoon sherry vinegar

½ cup chicken stock, preferably low sodium

Before You Start   The technique will work with any small whole bird prepared as detailed below, or even with bone-in chicken breasts. So-called game hens, which usually weigh about one pound each, will also work well here, although there is nothing remotely wild about a game hen; it's simply a small version of a regular chicken. Your quail should come with the backbone already cut out; to prepare a game hen to cook in the same way, see the Tip on page 145.

1. Clip the birds' wing tips off at the second joint down and discard or save for stock. Lay the birds out flat, skin side up, and pat them dry. Finely mince 10 of the sage leaves. Coarsely chop the remaining 10 leaves and set them aside. Rub the flattened birds all over with the smashed garlic and then with the finely minced sage. Season with the salt and a few grinds of pepper. Discard the smashed garlic.

2. Set two large, heavy-bottomed skillets or sauté pans over medium-high heat, and add 2 tablespoons of the olive oil to each. (You should be able to fit four quail or one game hen in each pan.) When the olive oil is very hot, add the birds skin side down. Cook without moving until the skin is dark golden brown and crisp.

- For quail, this should take about 7–8 minutes. Turn them and cook briefly on the other side, 3–4 minutes until cooked through. An instant-read thermometer should read 165°F.
- For game hens, place a heavy pan such as a cast-iron skillet or a saucepan weighted with a large can on top of the birds to encourage browning. Cook for about 15–20 minutes. Turn the

birds over and cook them on the other side (without a weight on top) for another 5–7 minutes, until cooked through per the temperature above.

3. Remove the birds to a serving platter and scrape any good crusty bits from one pan into the other. Set that pan over medium heat. Melt the butter in the pan until foamy, and then add the coarsely chopped sage leaves. Cook, stirring, for 1 minute, and then add the sherry vinegar. Cook for another minute, stirring. Add the chicken stock to the pan and simmer for 4–5 minutes, stirring to scrape up all the brown bits. Adjust seasoning to taste and serve the birds with the sauce.

From the Archives: By 1895, Shelburne Farms was home to more than two thousand farm-raised quail, which roamed free on the property, providing ample supplies for hunting forays. The *Burlington Farmers Advocate* noted the large flock and wryly observed, "It is hoped that this gamey little bird may thrive and luxuriate elsewhere than on toast"—in reference to a common recipe of the times, served at Shelburne House and elsewhere, in which small game birds were broiled and served on toast.

Tip: *To flatten a game hen, you will need to cut the backbone out with sharp kitchen scissors or poultry shears. Start at one side of the tail end (the little knobby piece) of the bird and cut straight down the back to the neck opening. Then repeat on the other side of the tail. (Discard the backbones or save them for stock.) Open the game hen like a book, turn it over, and press down on the breastbone firmly to flatten the bird. You now have a "spatchcocked" bird.*

Juniper and Maple Venison Steaks

Rick was inspired by New York City chef Gray Kunz to combine the aromatic forest scent of juniper and the sweetness of maple into a marinade and sauce for some stunningly dark red–purple venison steaks. It makes sense that the flavors marry well, as Vermont deer spend much of their time browsing evergreens and maple trees. Maple-Roasted Butternut Squash Puree and Soup (page 202) and Maple-Braised Red Cabbage with Pear and Cranberries (page 46) both go very well with this dish. ◇ **Serves: 4–6**

12 juniper berries, crushed medium-fine in a mortar and pestle or a spice grinder

1½ tablespoons gin

3 tablespoons pure maple syrup

1½ teaspoons coarse kosher salt plus more to taste

1 fresh rosemary sprig (4 inches long)

1½ pounds venison steaks, cut ¾ inch thick (see Before You Start)

1 tablespoon unsalted butter

Before You Start   Ask your butcher—or your favorite local hunter—for steaks cut from the top round, the top part of which is sometimes called the Denver leg. This recipe will also work with buffalo or bison steaks, which have the same deep but lean meatiness. Never cook venison or buffalo beyond medium-rare, as it will dry out and become tough. As Hank Dimuzio, a venison farmer from Middlebury says, "If you like well-done meat, do not eat venison. It's too lean."

1. In a shallow dish that will fit the steaks in one layer, whisk together the juniper berries, gin, maple syrup, and 1 teaspoon of the salt. Crush the rosemary sprig in your fist and add it to the marinade.

2. Place the venison steaks in the marinade and rub them with the rosemary sprig. Refrigerate the steaks for 1 hour, turning them halfway through. (Do not let them marinate longer or the alcohol will begin to change the texture of the meat.)

3. Prepare a barbecue grill to cook with medium-high heat. Alternatively, place a large broiler-proof skillet, preferably cast iron, on the oven rack in the second-highest slot, about 4–5 inches from the heating element. Preheat the broiler on its highest setting for at least 15 minutes.

4. Remove the steaks from the marinade, pat them dry, and remove any rosemary leaves. Reserve the marinade. Season the steaks with the remaining ½ teaspoon of salt on both sides.

5. Grill or broil the steaks for about 4–5 minutes per side for good color and a medium-rare interior. An instant-read thermometer should register about 140°F. While the steaks are cooking, pour the excess marinade into a small saucepan and bring it to a boil over medium-high heat. Take the pan off the heat and swirl in the butter. Let the steaks rest for at least 5 minutes after cooking, slice them very thin across the grain, and serve them drizzled with the sauce.

Keeping Tradition
Frank and Steve Leffler,
hunters

"I like to sit and watch the squirrels and the birds. I'm out with Mother Nature, being in the weather and the leaves coming down in all their colors."—Frank Leffler

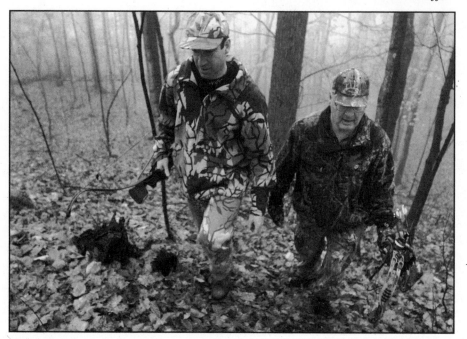

*h*unting is usually a passion handed down from father to son, but in the case of the Leffler family, it happened the other way around.

Steve was like most boys growing up in rural Vermont. "I got a shotgun when I was ten . . . and after school I would get my gun and hunt from my house to my friend's house, getting grouse, squirrels, rabbits," he recalls. "My dad took me deer hunting a few times and I loved it, but he wasn't really an avid hunter."

"Steve's been an outdoorsman from the beginning," says his father, Frank. In that, the two definitely share a passion. "I love to be in the woods," says Frank, who as a youngster also hunted small game. "We ate them too. I had a grandmother who knew how to prepare them," he adds. But with a general store to run and a family to raise, there wasn't much time to spend in the woods.

As the years passed, Frank caught some of his son's enthusiasm for hunting—for the connection it fosters to nature, for its role in keeping the environment in balance, for the satisfaction of bringing one's own meat to the table. Seven years ago, the Lefflers were among the first to respond to Shelburne Farms' call for experienced bow hunters.

The Lefflers hunt with rifles too, but they both favor the bow. "It's so one on one," explains Frank. "With bow hunting, you have to be really close to the deer, so you have to be a really good hunter. You have to be quiet and attentive. I love the challenge of it . . . I like to sit and watch the squirrels and the birds. I'm out with Mother Nature, being in the weather and the leaves coming down in all their colors."

Every fall at Shelburne Farms, Frank and Steve carefully scout their terrain on Butternut Hill to position their portable tree stands. "It's solo while you're sitting, but you track together," explains Steve. "I love the camaraderie of the hunt," says his dad, "the excitement of picking him up at four thirty in the morning. It keeps us close."

Early one misty fall morning, they start in an open field by an old wild apple tree where deer might gather to eat the fruit. The air is damp and cool. Walking from the field toward the edge of the woods, Steve points out the distinctive browse line the deer create, a remarkably precise line about five feet high, below which much of the young, tender growth has been stripped. It's better than it was when the pair began hunting at Shelburne Farms, but it's still a problem. "The deer can eat so much of the undergrowth, no new trees will grow," Frank explains.

Deep in the woods a few minutes later, copper and bronze leaves crunch softly underfoot. Steve stops to pick up an acorn. "This is the reason it's good hunting here," he says. "These are like deer candy." His dad holds out two similar-looking leaves from a red oak and a white oak. Deer will search out the sweeter acorns of a white oak, he explains; a good hunter will use that knowledge.

Raindrops are falling softly by the time they reach Steve's tree stand. He gestures up to the portable metal seat attached to a tall tree and says, "I solve all my life problems up there. I let my thoughts go where they want. One of the reasons I love bow hunting is it's really quiet." That is good for the deer too, he adds. "If you make a good shot, it's one hundred percent likely to kill, and with the bow, they don't even know what happened. They basically pass out, it's so quiet and sharp." No deer in the state of Vermont is going to die of old age, Steve continues. Most will be killed by cars, predators, disease, or starvation during long, cold winters. "One of the ways they can die is to be hit by a bow hunter's arrow. It's not a bad way to die, and the hunter is going to make full use of it."

Despite the fact that hunting is still very much a part of Vermont culture, it is no longer as intrinsic as it once was. Steve's son and daughter sometimes join their father and grandfather, but like most kids today, they juggle busy schedules of academics, sports, and other activities. "When I was in high school, in homeroom on Monday morning everyone wanted to know who got a deer over the weekend. Now my son doesn't even want to mention it," says Steve.

"The tradition of hunting is going away," concedes Frank. "For youngsters today, if you sit in a tree for three or four days without seeing a deer, you kind of lose their interest. It's too bad. It helps build a great love of the outdoors, the experience of really being in the wilderness and paying attention to what nature has to tell you. It's heritage and tradition . . . and it's wonderful table fare."

Venison Medallions with Cranberry Sauce

Few people are aware that there are Vermont-grown cranberries, and their season matches perfectly with the fall hunt—just as their deep red color and bright tart flavor go well with venison. ◇ **Serves: 4–6**

3 tablespoons olive oil

1½ pounds venison loin medallions, sliced ½ inch thick

2 teaspoons coarse kosher salt plus more to taste

3 small shallots, finely minced (about 3 tablespoons)

1 cup fruity red wine

1 cup fresh or frozen cranberries

2–3 tablespoons honey

2 tablespoons unsalted butter

Freshly ground black pepper to taste

Before You Start As in the previous venison recipe, buffalo or bison medallions would also work well here, and, once again, be careful never to cook venison beyond medium-rare. See Sources (page 273) for Vermont cranberries.

1. Set a large, heavy sauté pan or skillet over medium-high heat and add 2 tablespoons of the olive oil. Pat the venison dry and season on both sides with 1 teaspoon of the salt. Add the venison to the hot pan and cook without moving the meat until a nice golden brown crust develops, about 4 minutes per side. Do not overcook. Remove the venison to a plate and cover it loosely with foil to keep it warm.

2. Lower the heat to medium and add the remaining tablespoon of olive oil to the pan. Add the shallots and cook, stirring occasionally, until they are golden, 1–2 minutes.

3. Add the red wine and bring the sauce to a simmer, stirring to scrape up any brown bits. Add the cranberries to the pan and simmer about 5–7 minutes until the liquid is reduced and the cranberries have softened. Squish some of the cranberries with the back of a spoon or spatula.

4. Stir 2 tablespoons of honey into the sauce and cook for another minute. Take the pan off the heat and swirl the butter into the sauce. Add the remaining teaspoon of salt and black pepper to taste. Add more honey if desired. Serve the venison medallions drizzled with the sauce.

Venison Chili

Every hunter has a favorite chili recipe to simmer up on an old stove at deer camp. Chili lends itself perfectly to lean, flavorful venison meat. This version, deepened with the classic Mexican combination of cinnamon and chocolate, was inspired by a recipe from a local brew pub called Bobcat Café. Serve with shredded cheddar, a big green salad dressed with buttermilk dressing (from the Tip on page 25), and Streuseled Maple Corn Muffins (page 260) without the streusel. ◇ ***Serves: 4–6***

2 tablespoons olive oil

1 large onion, finely chopped (about 1½ cups)

4 cloves garlic, minced (about 1 tablespoon)

1 tablespoon chili powder

2 teaspoons ground cumin

1 teaspoon ground cinnamon

1 pound ground venison meat

2 tablespoons all-purpose flour

2 teaspoons unsweetened cocoa powder

1 (28-ounce) can diced tomatoes, preferably fire-roasted (see Before You Start)

1 cup dark Mexican beer (see Before You Start)

1 teaspoon dried oregano leaves, preferably Mexican

1 chipotle chili pepper in adobo sauce, finely chopped (see Before You Start)

2 (15.5-ounce) cans kidney beans or 1 can kidney beans and 1 can black beans, drained and rinsed

2 teaspoons coarse kosher salt plus more to taste

Freshly ground black pepper to taste

Before You Start   Lean ground beef, ground buffalo meat, or even ground turkey could be substituted for the venison. Fire-roasted canned tomatoes, such as those from Muir Glen, deepen the smoky flavor. Look for Dos Equis Amber or Negra Modelo beer, and you can find small cans of chipotle chili peppers in adobo sauce in the Mexican section of many supermarkets. They keep forever in the refrigerator (see Maple-Chipotle Scallops, page 47, for another use).

1. In a large, heavy-bottomed soup pot set over medium-high heat, heat the oil. Add the onion, garlic, chili powder, cumin, and cinnamon and sauté until the onion is soft, about 5–6 minutes.

2. Add the venison and cook, stirring occasionally to break up the meat, until it is browned, about 7–10 minutes.

3. Sprinkle in the flour and cocoa and cook, stirring, for another 2 minutes. Stir in the tomatoes, beer, oregano, and chipotle chili pepper.

4. Increase the heat to bring the chili to a simmer. Stir in the beans, salt, and a few grinds of black pepper. Simmer, uncovered, for about 20 minutes, stirring occasionally to prevent sticking. Adjust seasoning to taste and serve.

Prepare-Ahead Tip: *Chili can be made a few days ahead, kept in the refrigerator and reheated over a low flame, stirring to prevent sticking. It also freezes well.*

Cornmeal Fried Trout with Bacon and Sage

[photograph 13]

There's nothing like trout fried in a well-seasoned cast-iron skillet with some bacon fat. The honey-sage butter is a little different; it adds a lightly sweet, woodsy note to the fish and balances the salty bacon. Try this with Winter Root Slaw (page 195) and a puddle of grits made with the same stone-ground cornmeal used to coat the fish. ◇ Serves: 4

16 large fresh sage leaves

3 tablespoons unsalted butter, at room temperature

2 teaspoons honey

¾ cup yellow or white cornmeal, preferably stone-ground

1½ teaspoons baking powder

1 teaspoon coarse kosher salt

Freshly ground black pepper to taste

1 large egg white

2 teaspoons water

4 brook or rainbow trout fillets (6–8 ounces each)

6 pieces thick-cut bacon (about 6 ounces)

Before You Start   The baking powder whisked in with the cornmeal gives the fish a crisp coat—a tip from an old Vermont cookbook. We are lucky to have locally grown and ground heirloom flint corn. Look for stone-ground cornmeal in natural foods stores and in the baking aisle of some supermarkets; fine cornmeal works too, but won't deliver quite the same crunch.

1. Finely chop four of the sage leaves and mix with 1 tablespoon of the butter and the honey in a small bowl. Set aside.

2. Pour the cornmeal into a shallow, rimmed plate or pie pan and whisk in the baking powder, the salt, and a few grinds of pepper. In a second similar plate or pan, whisk the egg white with the water. Pat the trout dry and dip both sides of each fillet into the egg white mixture and then the cornmeal mixture to coat.

3. In a large sauté pan, or preferably a cast-iron skillet, cook the bacon until crisp and then set it aside on paper towel to drain. Pour off all but 2 tablespoons of the bacon fat and reserve. Add 1 tablespoon of the butter to the skillet. Heat over medium-high until the fat is sizzling.

4. Add the fish to the skillet, two fillets at a time, and fry until crisp, about 4 minutes on each side. As the fish comes hot out of the pan, scoop a little honey-sage butter onto each fillet so it melts into the hot crust. Cover the first batch loosely with foil while finishing the second batch.

5. Add a little more bacon fat and the remaining tablespoon of butter to the pan and fry the remaining fillets along with the remaining whole sage leaves, which should take just 1 minute to crisp and can be removed while the fillets finish cooking. Serve the trout topped with the fried sage leaves and crumbled bacon.

Prepare-Ahead Tip: *The honey-sage butter can be made a few days ahead and kept in the refrigerator.*

Whole Roast Trout with Ramps and Herbs

Ideally, you'd land your first-of-the-season brook trout and then gather ramps (wild leeks), watercress, or garlic mustard in and around the same rushing stream, chilly with snowmelt, to create a fully wild meal. But you can also gather the fish, along with scallions and an array of soft green herbs, at your market instead.

◇ *Serves: 4*

12 ramps or large scallions with tops as long as possible, roots trimmed

1 tablespoon plus 2 teaspoons olive oil

4 whole brook or rainbow trout, 8–10 ounces each, preferably butterflied (see Before You Start)

1½ teaspoons coarse kosher salt

Freshly ground black pepper to taste

8 sprigs each of any 3–4 of the following: wild greens such as watercress or garlic mustard, flat-leaf parsley, dill, chives, tarragon, chervil, fennel fronds

1 lemon, washed well, one half sliced into 8 thin rounds, the other half wedged to serve with the fish

Spring Herb Mayonnaise (page 63) made with the herbs used to stuff the trout

Before You Start Although the widely available farmed trout can reach up to a pound apiece, look for whole trout that are not more than ten ounces dressed weight. If possible, you want your trout butterflied, which means it is gutted and boned without the head and the two fillets are still attached along the back. Clip off the fins with kitchen shears. If the bones are still in the fish, just eat around them. Be careful choosing your pan, as some ovenproof skillets are not up to the high heat of the broiler.

1. Place a large broilerproof skillet, preferably cast iron, on the oven rack in the second-highest position, about 4–5 inches from the heating element. Preheat the broiler on its highest setting for at least 15 minutes.

2. Take eight of the ramps and cut off but reserve the top 2–3 inches of the greens. Put the trimmed ramps on a plate and drizzle with 2 teaspoons of the olive oil. Set aside.

3. Pat the trout dry inside and out and brush each trout with the remaining olive oil on both sides before seasoning well with the salt and a few grinds of pepper outside and in. Put two sprigs of each herb, plus two of the trimmed ramp tops, into each fish cavity. Lay two lemon rounds in each one.

4. Take the remaining four ramps and cut the bulbs from the greens. Put one bulb into each fish cavity. Using the full length of the remaining greens, tie each trout around its middle with the greens in a loose knot.

5. Carefully open the oven and lay the stuffed trout on the preheated (and very hot!) skillet. Toss the eight olive oil-drizzled ramps into the skillet around the fish. With the oven door slightly ajar, broil the trout for 7–9 minutes until the skin is crisp and the fish is cooked through. The ramps should be lightly charred. The ones tying the trout may burn through, but they have served their purpose and can be discarded.

6. Serve each trout immediately with a generous dollop of Spring Herb Mayonnaise and lemon wedges.

> **Prepare-Ahead Tip:** *The Spring Herb Mayonnaise can be made a few days ahead and kept in the refrigerator.*

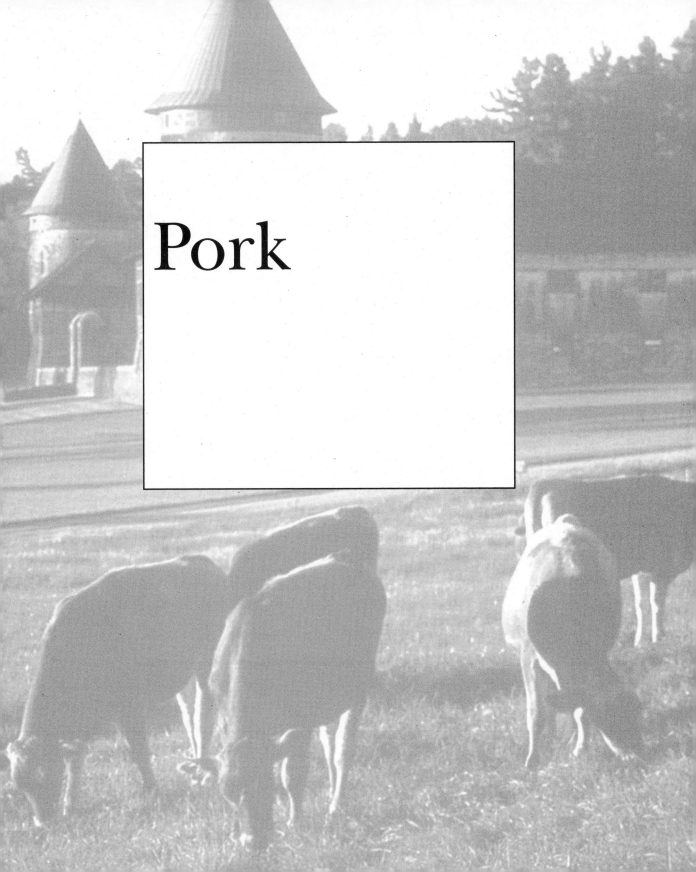

Pork

- Ham and Cantaloupe Chopped Salad
- Bacon and Goat Cheese Free-Form Tart
- Deviled Ham and Cheddar Spread
- Sausage Rolls
- Maple-Glazed Ribs
- Roast Chicken with Sausages and Apples
- Ale-Braised Kielbasa with Sauerkraut
- Crispy Pork Chops with Parsley Sauce
- Pork Loin with Pear and Cornbread Stuffing
- Slow-Roasted Pork Shoulder with Fennel and Orange

*i*n a steeply sloping field behind the Farm Barn at Shelburne Farms, a pen of corkscrew-tailed piglets starts each season playing musical teats at the belly of their giant, long-suffering mother. The sow and her litter are on an extended visit from Duclos and Thompson Farm, about twenty-five miles south of Shelburne. As the piglets grow, they jostle over tasty Market-Garden vegetable scraps and whey left from cheesemaking, making their contribution to recycling on the Farm. Small visitors giggle as they watch the piglets try to stay cool in the summer sun, snorting and pushing each other out of coveted patches of mud and shade.

Back in Vermont's subsistence farming days of the early 1800s, a hog or two was an important part of the self-sufficiency loop. They greedily snuffled up kitchen leftovers and other edible farmyard scraps until late fall, when they were slaughtered for the year ahead. Almost every bit of the animal was used: lard was destined for piecrusts, head cheese was made from the head, intestines became sausage casings. Bacon and hams were cured in smokehouses over corncobs—another thrifty New England practice—and the salty, smoky flavor of cured pork broke up the monotony of cold-weather cooking. Pork in its many forms has always paired particularly well with other classic Vermont ingredients like maple and apples.

A model shingle-and-brick, dormered piggery was built at Shelburne Farms in 1897 with lots of room, light, and outdoor access for the animals. Farm hogs—fed on grain and skim milk from the dairy—were raised for the family and staff and also sold at market and to the Vanderbilt railroad network. The pork venture was actually started by fifteen-year-old Frederica, Lila and Seward Webb's only daughter, to show her business ability and to earn a little extra spending money. It proved so profitable, however, a local newspaper reported that, after a few years, "Dr. Webb thought it advisable to buy her out."

As transportation options increased, farmers shipped pork by canal and by rail, and Vermont became known for its cob-smoked hams. While pork is no longer a significant part of the state's agricultural picture, Vermont smoked hams are still well regarded nationally, and independent food markets cobble together a supply of richly flavored, fresh and cured pork from a patchwork of small farms raising pigs alongside other animals.

A Note About Pork

The quality of pork has suffered from efforts over the last decade to reposition it as a lean "white" meat. This makes it even more important to search out smaller-scale, locally raised meat from animals that have room to grow and develop some of the fat and flavor we've lost in commercial pork. Although some cuts, like tenderloin and some chops, will always be fairly lean, in most cases you want to see some fat.

To compensate for the lack of fat, much fresh supermarket pork is now injected with a salt solution to replace the moisture and flavor previously provided by fat. It is often called "enhanced" pork. Check the label, and if that's all you can find, decrease added salt to allow for this.

One thing that's changed for the better is that the parasitic disease trichinosis has been virtually eliminated from the national pork supply, so it is no longer necessary to cook pork until gray to ensure food safety. It is still important to measure the internal temperature of the meat, mostly when cooking larger roasts, so please buy an instant-read meat thermometer if you don't yet have one. The U.S. Department of Agriculture now officially sanctions 160°F as a safe internal temperature for pork, but we would encourage you to consider taking leaner cuts, like the Pork Loin (page 179), from the oven at 145°F, knowing the temperature will climb a little as they rest. Yet another reason to know and trust the sources of your food.

Ham and Cantaloupe Chopped Salad

What's not to love about the well-matched trio of salty, meaty, dry-cured ham; sweet, ripe melon; and the creamy bite of crumbled blue cheese? The light licorice hint in the tarragon dressing brings an unexpected and refreshing touch to this perfect summer lunch or supper. For an extra touch, try a few Spiced Maple Nuts (page 41) sprinkled on top of the salad. ◇ **Makes: 4 main course salads**

For the salad

1 long English cucumber, no need to peel or seed, or 2 regular cucumbers, peeled and seeded

1 large heart of romaine lettuce

¾ pound best-quality, smoked ham (about 2½-inch thick slices)

½ medium cantaloupe, seeded and peeled

½ cup (about 2–3 ounces) crumbled best-quality blue cheese

For the dressing

½ cup sour cream

¼ cup buttermilk (see Tips, pages 25 and 163)

1 tablespoon freshly squeezed lemon juice

2 tablespoons finely sliced fresh tarragon leaves

1 tablespoon medium dry sherry or apple juice

½ teaspoon coarse kosher salt plus more to taste

Freshly ground black pepper to taste

Before You Start   Go for the best smoked ham you can find. We have some great ones in Vermont (see Sources, page 273), but any good Black Forest-style, dry-cured ham will work. This salad will also shine with a really good blue cheese. See page 116 for some of our favorite Vermont blue cheeses. Try to avoid those packages of pre-crumbled, dried-out nuggets.

1. Cut the cucumber, lettuce, ham, and cantaloupe into ½-inch dice. Toss together in a large bowl.

2. In a small bowl, whisk together the sour cream, buttermilk, lemon juice, tarragon, sherry, and salt. Adjust seasoning to taste.

3. Right before serving, pour the dressing over the salad and toss gently. Serve topped with the crumbled blue cheese.

From the Archives: In the early 1900s, the Shelburne Farms gardener cultivated a variety of melons, including the green-fleshed Bay View Musk melon, the Sweet Siberian watermelon with golden flesh, and the translucent white Hero of Lockinge, a melon named for the man who founded the British Red Cross. The range of color and texture must have been impressive, as the melons merited their own course at no less an event than a prewedding celebration hosted at Shelburne House a few days before Vanderbilt Webb's marriage in 1912. The first course on the elaborate menu is simply "Shelburne Farms melons," followed by Green Turtle Soup.

Tip: *In dressings that call for buttermilk, plain yogurt thinned with water makes a decent substitute. Measure out ¾ of the called-for quantity of yogurt and whisk in water to make up the balance.*

Pork

Bacon and Goat Cheese Free-Form Tart

[photograph 14]

The cornmeal in the crust adds a nutty crunch and complements the smoky, salty bacon and fresh goat cheese. The tart makes a perfect light lunch or supper with a green salad. ◇ *Serves: 4 as a main course, 8 as an appetizer*

For the crust

½ cup (1 stick) unsalted butter, cold

1¼ cup all-purpose flour

¼ cup yellow or white cornmeal, preferably stone-ground

½ teaspoon coarse kosher salt

3 ounces cream cheese, cold and cut into 4 chunks

2–3 tablespoons ice water

Milk to brush the crust

For the filling

8 slices thick-cut bacon (about ½ pound)

1 tablespoon olive oil

2 pounds (about 4 large) onions, thinly sliced

½ teaspoon coarse kosher salt

1 teaspoon fresh thyme leaves

¾ cup (3–4 ounces) crumbled fresh goat cheese

Before You Start   We use locally grown and ground heirloom flint corn. Look for stone-ground cornmeal in natural foods stores and in the baking aisle of some supermarkets; fine cornmeal works too, but won't deliver quite the same crunch.

1. *Make the crust:* Cut the butter into small cubes and freeze for at least 15 minutes.

2. In the bowl of a food processor fitted with the metal blade, blend the flour, cornmeal, and salt. Add the cream cheese and process for about 20 seconds, or until the mixture resembles coarse crumbs. Add the butter and pulse until no butter is larger than the size of a pea. Add the ice water and process for about 30 seconds, or until a pinch of the dough holds together. If it doesn't, add more water, a teaspoon at a time.

3. Dump the dough out onto a lightly floured counter. Knead just until it holds together in one piece. Shape the dough into a flat disk, wrap it in plastic wrap, and refrigerate it for at least 30 minutes. (If you chill it much longer, give it time to warm up a little before rolling it out.)

4. *Make the filling:* While the dough is chilling, cook the bacon in a sauté pan or skillet until it is about halfway cooked. Remove the bacon to a plate lined with paper towel and set aside.

5. Discard all but 2 tablespoons of the bacon fat. Put the pan with the remaining bacon fat back over medium heat. Add the olive oil and then the sliced onions and salt. Reduce the heat to medium-low and cook the onions slowly, stirring occasionally, until they are deep golden brown and caramelized, 35–45 minutes.

6. Preheat the oven to 375°F with a rack in the second-lowest position. On a nonstick baking mat or piece of parchment paper, roll the chilled dough into a rough circle about ⅛ inch thick and 14–16 inches in diameter. (The edges do not have to be smooth and neat.) Lift the baking mat with the crust onto a cookie sheet.

7. Spread the caramelized onions over the crust, leaving a ½-inch border around the edge. Coarsely chop the bacon and sprinkle it evenly over the onions, followed by the thyme leaves, and finally the goat cheese. Fold the edges of the crust in over the filling, pleating the edges as necessary. Brush the crust with milk.

8. Bake the tart for about 30–35 minutes until the crust is golden. Serve hot, warm, or at room temperature.

Variation The onion and bacon base also works well with cooked diced beets; raw diced apple; and blue cheese. Or substitute diced ham for the bacon and add lightly steamed or microwaved cubes of butternut squash or pumpkin and goat cheese. Skip the bacon for a vegetarian tart.

Prepare-Ahead Tip: *The caramelized onions and the crust (unrolled) can be stored for a week in the refrigerator. The crust can also be frozen and thawed in the refrigerator overnight. Give the crust a little time to warm up before rolling it out. The tart can be assembled on the cookie sheet, loosely covered with plastic wrap, and refrigerated for up to twelve hours. Bring it to room temperature before baking.*

Teaching Pigs to Sing

Lisa Thompson and Tom Duclos, farmers, Duclos and Thompson Farm

"They're smart. They're creative. They're resourceful. If a pig has an itch on its butt, it'll figure out how to scratch it."—Lisa Thompson

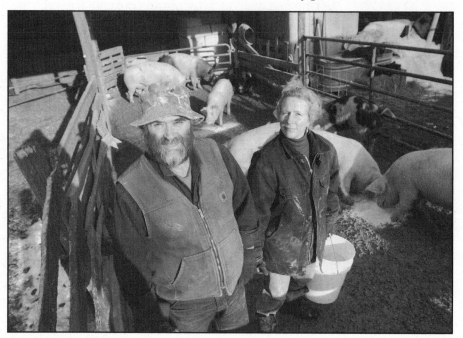

"Never try to teach a pig to sing," reads a sign hanging in the barn at Duclos and Thompson Farm in Weybridge. "It wastes your time and annoys the pig."

Husband and wife Tom Duclos and Lisa Thompson have run their small, diversified farm together for twenty-five years. They started with sheep—and lambs still make up about a third of their business—but about twenty years ago Tom brought home a couple of pigs from auction. Lisa was not too pleased when her husband arrived with the two pregnant sows. "I didn't think I wanted anything to do with them. I thought they were dirty, smelly animals," she recalls.

"I knew she didn't care for them, but I figured if one showed up here, she'd get used to it," her husband says with a mischievous grin. He was right. "It was a big misconception," she admits, smiling back at him. "They're smart. They're creative. They're resourceful. If a pig has an itch on its butt, it'll figure out how to scratch it." Their love of mud may be seen as dirty, she explains, but it is actually a pig's way of staying cool because the animals have no sweat glands.

The couple now raises close to three hundred pigs a year, which they sell to independent food markets and restaurants, and direct to devoted customers who trek to the farm to pick up ribs, chops, or smoked bacon from a small self-serve farm stand. It's the old-fashioned kind of pork, not afraid to show its fat.

Since they started selling pork eight years ago, it has grown to a third of the farm's earnings, and is Duclos and Thompson's only year-round business. "It's the first time we've ever had a regular income," observes Lisa. To make ends meet, Tom drives trucks for a feed company a few days a week in exchange for livestock feed, and the couple does custom work like haying other farms during the summer or loaning pigs out to Shelburne Farms. When they deliver pork to one of their major restaurant customers, they pick up the kitchen's vegetable scraps to feed to the next set of pigs. Diversity has been key to keeping the farm going. "The theory is that they don't all lose money at the same time," says Tom wryly.

Things have changed, Tom reflects as he stands in front of a pen of three-month-old pigs huddled together for companionship and warmth on a chilly winter day. ("You've heard of a hog pile?" he says.) Nodding his head to the south out over a snowy field, he indicates where he grew up on a farm a few miles away. After his father died, his mother supported the three (of seven) children left at home with eggs from a hundred chickens and butter and cream from about fifteen cows. "Couldn't do that today," he says.

Like so many small Vermont farmers, Tom and Lisa can't imagine doing anything else. "I'm better with animals than people," says Lisa. "I'm just a farmer," Tom shrugs. It helps that they're also smart, creative, and resourceful—just like their pigs.

Deviled Ham and Cheddar Spread

[photograph 21]

This spread is a great way to use up bits of leftover ham and cheddar cheese. It was inspired by the sandwich fillings served at the Inn for afternoon tea. Try topping it with thin slices of apple, or spread it thickly on a nice, crusty piece of bread and pop it in the toaster oven until it's bubbly. For a quick appetizer, fill celery stalks with it or dollop it in the center of cucumber slices and then dust with more paprika for color. ◊ **Makes: 1½ cups sandwich spread (can easily be doubled)**

½ cup (2 ounces) grated cheddar

1 cup (4 ounces) roughly chopped best-quality smoked ham

3 tablespoons mayonnaise

1 tablespoon Dijon mustard

1 small dill pickle (about 3 inches long) plus pickle juice to thin spread if needed

3 dashes hot pepper sauce, such as Tabasco, plus more to taste

⅛ teaspoon sweet paprika

Before You Start   A nice, sharp, aged cheddar like Shelburne Farms one- or two-year works well here. Start with the coarse grating disc in your food processor to grate the cheese, then switch to the blade to make the spread. See Before You Start on page 162 for more information on smoked hams.

1. Combine the cheddar, ham, mayonnaise, mustard, dill pickle, hot pepper sauce, and paprika in the bowl of a food processor and pulse to combine, but don't make the spread completely smooth. Add a little pickle juice if the spread seems too thick.

2. Taste and add more hot pepper sauce if desired. The spread keeps for two or three days in the refrigerator.

Variation   Rick also uses this spread to make super deviled eggs. He adds the soft egg yolks to the spread along with a little more mayonnaise. See The Whole-Pea Salad with Deviled Farm Barn Eggs (page 68) for the perfect hard-cooked egg method.

Sausage Rolls

These are a taste I remember fondly from my English childhood, when we'd often eat them on excursions to grand country estates reminiscent of Shelburne Farms. The touch of nutmeg and clove in the pork filling also echoes the French-Canadian meat pies that have become a part of Vermont's food culture. They make perfect picnic fare and go especially well with pickles like our Pickled Ramps (page 59) or Quick Pickled Carrots and Rutabagas (page 189). You could also make smaller, bite-size versions for parties. ◇ ***Makes: twelve 3-inch sausage rolls***

1 (17.3-ounce) box frozen puff pastry (two 10 by 10-inch sheets)

2 large eggs

1 pound lean ground pork

1 cup soft, fresh bread crumbs

1 small onion, finely minced

2 cloves garlic, finely minced

2 tablespoons minced fresh flat-leaf parsley

2 tablespoons minced fresh thyme leaves

1 tablespoon Dijon mustard

¼ teaspoon ground nutmeg

¼ teaspoon ground cloves

1 teaspoon coarse kosher salt

½ teaspoon freshly ground black pepper

1 tablespoon water

Before You Start   If you can custom-order your ground pork, ask for it lean. If your pork is ground from trimmings of the brine-injected "enhanced" pork found in many supermarkets today, use only ½ teaspoon salt.

1. Thaw the puff pastry according to the package directions. Preheat the oven to 400°F with racks in the second and third positions from the bottom. Lightly grease two cookie sheets and set them aside.

2. In a large mixing bowl, beat one of the eggs and then add the pork, bread crumbs, onion, garlic, parsley, thyme, mustard, nutmeg, cloves, salt, and pepper. Mix well with a spoon or with your hands.

3. Unfold the first sheet of puff pastry onto one of the prepared cookie sheets and cut it into two even pieces. Take one quarter of the pork filling and make a 2-inch-wide tube of it down the length of one of the pieces, reaching the edge of the pastry at each end but leaving about 1½ inches on either side. Do the same with the second half of that puff pastry sheet and another quarter of the filling.

4. In a small bowl, beat the remaining egg with the water. Fold one side of the puff pastry up over the filling. Brush the top of the pastry you have just folded with egg wash, and then brush the opposite edge with egg wash. Fold that second edge up over the filling to overlap its partner and press down gently to seal. Carefully flip the sausage roll over and slice it across into three even rolls, each roughly three inches long. Brush the tops with egg wash and cut two short diagonal slashes in each.

5. Repeat with the second sheet of puff pastry on the second cookie sheet.

6. Bake the sausage rolls for 15 minutes. Reduce the oven temperature to 350°F and swap the cookie sheets between the two racks. Bake for another 15 minutes or until the sausage rolls are puffed and golden brown. Serve warm or at room temperature with additional mustard.

Prepare-Ahead Tip: Although sausage rolls are best baked fresh, you can bake these a couple of days ahead and keep them in the refrigerator. You will want to eat them at room temperature or rewarmed to crisp up the pastry a little.

Maple-Glazed Ribs

[photograph 15]

Although Rick doesn't have much opportunity to serve ribs at the Inn, they are one of his favorite things to make for friends and family, and he is quite an expert on different styles of barbecue. He would slow-cook these in his kettle grill, but the oven makes them much easier and more predictable. This recipe makes a sweet, sticky rib—not the wet, sloppy kind. Red Cabbage, Pear, and Cranberry Slaw (page 43) makes a great side dish, as do Streuseled Maple Corn Muffins (page 260) without the streusel. ◇ ***Serves: 4–6***

2 tablespoons garlic powder

2½ tablespoons coarse kosher salt

1 tablespoon mustard powder, such as Colman's

3 packed tablespoons light brown sugar

2 tablespoons plus 1 teaspoon smoked sweet Spanish paprika or sweet paprika

4 pounds baby back ribs

½ cup beer, preferably an amber ale (see Before You Start)

½ cup maple syrup, Grade B for strongest flavor

¼ cup cider vinegar

¼ cup ketchup

Before You Start Ideally, you would rub the ribs ahead of time and let them absorb the flavors for at least an hour, but the recipe works well even without doing that. Using smoked sweet Spanish paprika brings a wonderful smokiness to these ribs, but they will be delicious with regular paprika too. You can find smoked sweet paprika in some specialty markets, or see Sources, page 273. We like Vermont's Long Trail amber ale in the mop—and to drink with the ribs too.

1. Preheat the oven to 325°F. In a small bowl, whisk together the garlic powder, salt, mustard powder, brown sugar, and 2 tablespoons of the paprika. Set aside about 1½ tablespoons of the rub, and rub the rest over both sides of the ribs.

2. With the meaty side down, wrap each rack of ribs in foil like a package. Place them on a rimmed cookie sheet or shallow roasting pan. Cook for about 2 hours until the meat is very tender.

3. Increase the oven temperature to 450°F with a rack in the second-highest position. Unwrap the ribs carefully, pour off and discard any accumulated fat, and replace the ribs on the foil in the pan.

4. In a small saucepan, whisk together the beer, maple syrup, and cider vinegar. Using a basting brush or crumpled paper towel, mop both sides of the ribs well with the mixture, finishing with the meaty side up. Reserve the remaining mop.

5. Sprinkle the reserved rub over the meaty side of the ribs and cook them in the oven for about 10 minutes until glazed and crusty.

6. While the ribs are finishing, whisk the remaining 1 teaspoon of paprika and the ketchup into the reserved mop. Simmer it over medium heat for 5–7 minutes until slightly thickened. Adjust seasoning to taste and serve with the ribs.

Roast Chicken with Sausages and Apples

Few things can improve upon a perfect roast chicken, but adding nice, fat, browned sausages and soft, caramelized apple slices definitely brings something to the party. My English aunt gets credit for introducing me to roast chicken with sausages. Rick likes to toast pieces of crusty, country-style bread, cube them, and then toss them in the pan drippings (before making the cider gravy) to serve with the chicken. ◇ *Serves: 4–6*

1 chicken, about 4½ pounds

1½ teaspoons coarse kosher salt plus more to taste

2 tablespoons olive oil

1½ tablespoons freshly squeezed lemon juice

1 pound fat pork sausages (see Before You Start), cut into 2-inch lengths

5 large shallots, peeled and trimmed with the root end left intact so that they can be cut in half and hold together

3 large, firm apples such as Empire, Macoun, Northern Spy, or Gala, cored but not peeled, each cut into 8 wedges

16 large fresh sage leaves

¾ cup apple cider

Before You Start   Since you will also be serving sausages, you can go with a slightly smaller chicken than you might normally roast. The classic pudgy, mildly seasoned, English banger–style sausages are not always easy to find here, but a simple breakfast sausage or bratwurst works. If they're breakfast sausage-size rather than bratwurst-size, leave the sausages whole.

1. Preheat the oven to 400°F with a rack in the lowest position. Carefully slide your fingers under the chicken breast skin and gently separate the skin from the flesh. Rub the breast meat under the skin with 1 teaspoon of the salt. Rub the outer skin of the chicken all over with the olive oil and lemon juice and season with the remaining salt.

2. Set the chicken on a low rack in a large roasting pan. Roast for 30 minutes.

3. Reduce the oven temperature to 375°F. Add the sausages, shallots, apples, and sage to the pan around the chicken and toss in the pan juices, adding a little olive oil if the pan seems too dry. Roast for another 45–55 minutes, turning the sausages, shallots, and apples once, until the chicken is golden brown and an instant-read thermometer inserted into the chicken thigh registers 175°F. Set the chicken on a carving board to rest. Scoop the sausages, shallots, and apples into a serving bowl and cover to keep warm. (Don't worry about the sage leaves—they can be wherever they please.)

4. Set the roasting pan over two burners on medium heat. Bring the drippings to a simmer and add the apple cider, stirring and scraping up any brown bits. Simmer for 2–3 minutes. Adjust seasoning to taste.

5. Carve the chicken and serve with pieces of sausage, shallots, and apples on the side and the cider-sage gravy passed at the table.

Ale-Braised Kielbasa with Sauerkraut

Rick makes this earthy, comforting dish for his mountain biking buddies. Serve it on a chilly day with a side of Oven-Roasted Applesauce (page 229).

◇ *Serves: 6–8*

2–3 tablespoons olive oil

2 pounds smoked pork kielbasa or smoked pork and beef kielbasa, each 1-pound coil cut into 6 equal lengths

5 cloves garlic, smashed with the flat side of a knife

1 small onion, halved, and thinly sliced crosswise

1 cup brown ale (see Before You Start)

1 cup apple cider or natural apple juice

2 sprigs fresh rosemary

2 pounds all-purpose potatoes, such as Yukon gold, not peeled, well scrubbed, and cut into 1-inch chunks

1 teaspoon coarse kosher salt plus more to taste

3 cups sauerkraut, drained and rinsed if desired

Before You Start   We find we don't need to rinse the wonderful local sauerkraut we use, but if you buy the more commercial stuff or don't love the briny flavor, you may want to. You can use any beer with some flavor, but brown ale's malty sweetness balances the rich kielbasa and sauerkraut best. In Vermont we like Wolaver's Brown Ale or Long Trail Double Bag Ale. The classic English Newcastle Brown Ale is quite widely available.

1. Preheat the oven to 350°F. In a large ovenproof skillet set over medium-high heat, heat the olive oil until hot. Add the kielbasa pieces, in batches if necessary so as not to crowd, and cook, turning, until just starting to color. Add more oil if needed. When all the kielbasa is lightly browned, put it all back in the pan and lower the heat to medium. Add the garlic cloves and sliced onion and continue cooking, stirring occasionally, until the onion is golden and the kielbasa is deeply browned, about 10–12 minutes.

2. Remove the kielbasa to a plate. Pour the ale and apple cider into the pan, add the rosemary, and increase the heat to medium-high. Simmer for 8–10 minutes until the liquid is reduced by about half.

3. Add the potatoes and sprinkle with the salt. Cover and simmer for 10 minutes. Stir in the sauerkraut and return the kielbasa to the pan.

Pork

4. Cover with a lid or foil and bake in the oven for 35–40 minutes until the potatoes are cooked through. Remove the rosemary sprigs and adjust seasoning to taste. Serve with stone-ground mustard and applesauce if desired.

Variation If you don't like sauerkraut, try this recipe with 4 cups of shredded green cabbage instead.

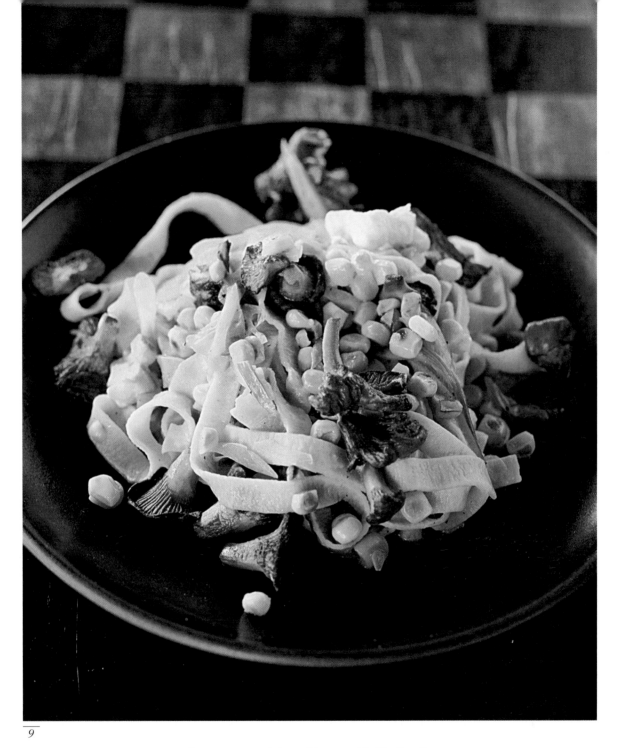

Chanterelles, Corn, and Goat Cheese with Tagliatelle *(page 111)*

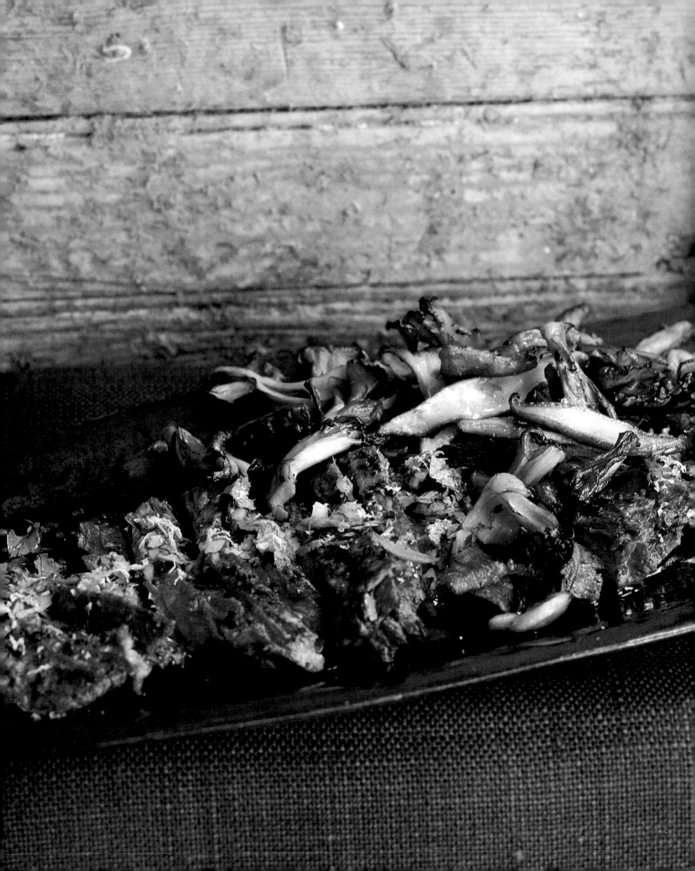

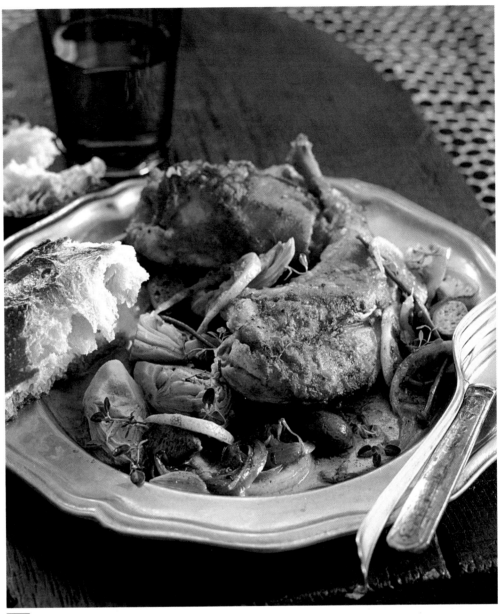

Braised Rabbit with Artichokes, Capers, and Lemon *(page 136)*

Opposite: Grilled Steak with
Cumin-Coriander Mushrooms
(page 128)

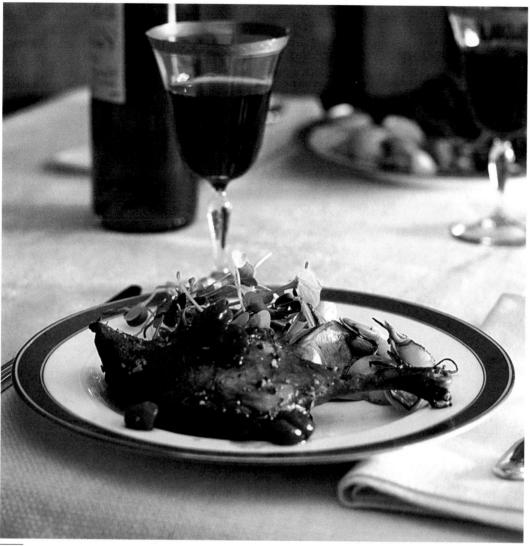

Roast Duck Legs with Sour Cherry Sauce *(page 142)*
with Honey-Glazed Turnips *(page 197)*

Opposite: Cornmeal Fried Trout with
Bacon and Sage *(page 153)* with Winter
Root Slaw *(page 195)*

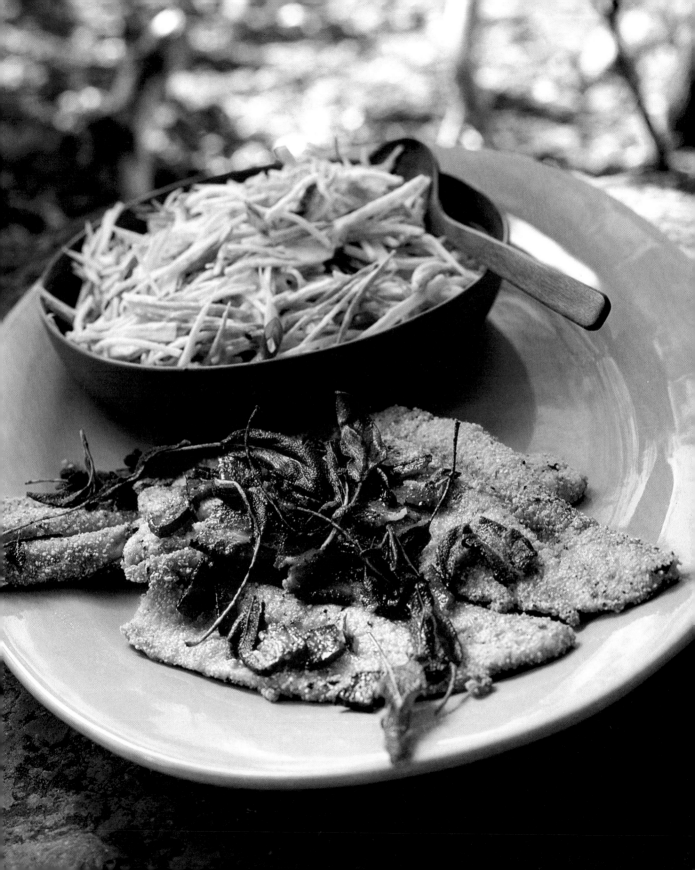

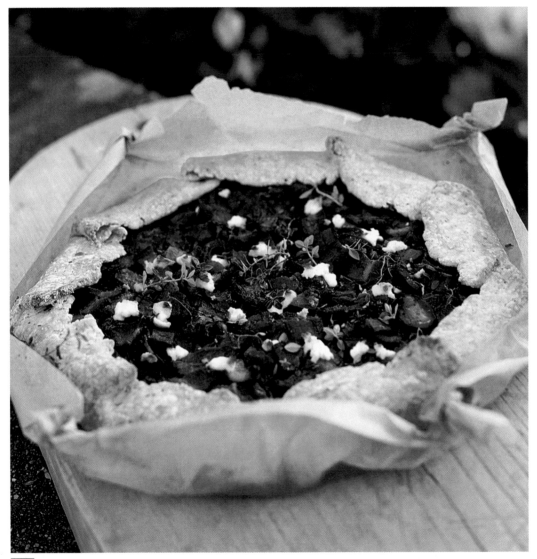

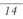

Bacon and Goat Cheese Free-Form Tart *(page 164)*

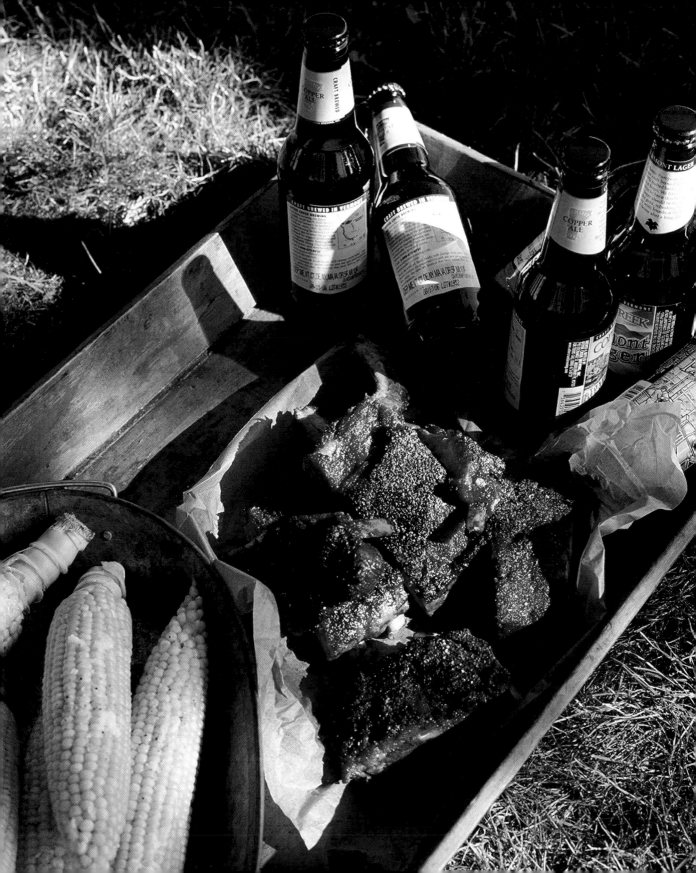

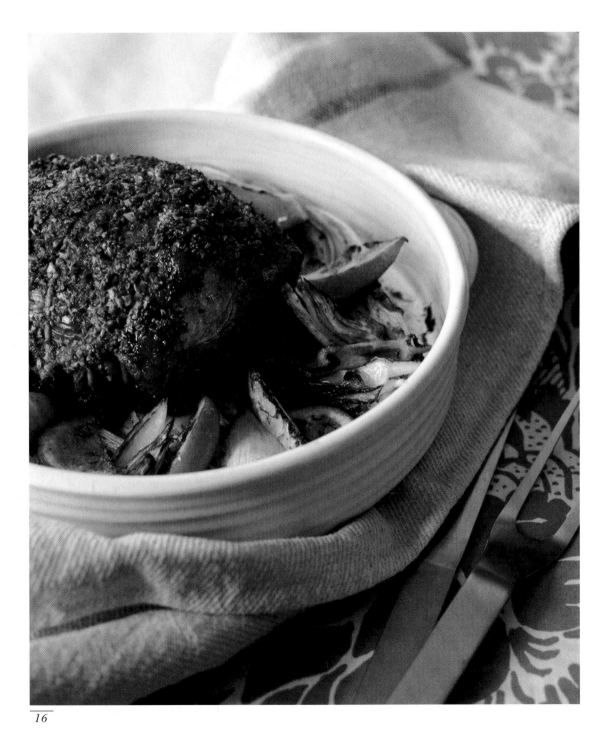

Slow-Roasted Pork Shoulder with Fennel and Orange *(page 181)*

Crispy Pork Chops with Parsley Sauce

This classic schnitzel preparation with pork is spiced up with a little coriander and cumin and then brightened with a parsley and lemon sauce. It makes a great, quick weeknight family supper. Don't skip the sauce; it really makes the dish. ◇ *Serves: 4*

For the sauce

3 tablespoons freshly squeezed lemon juice (see Tip, page 75)

¼ teaspoon ground cumin

¼ teaspoon ground coriander

½ teaspoon coarse kosher salt plus more to taste

¼ cup olive oil

½ cup finely chopped fresh flat-leaf parsley

2 large shallots, finely minced, or ¼ cup finely minced red onion

For the pork

¼ cup all-purpose flour

2 large eggs

1½ cups coarse bread crumbs, fresh or dry

1 teaspoon ground coriander

1 teaspoon ground cumin

1 teaspoon coarse kosher salt

Freshly ground black pepper to taste

¼ cup olive oil

8 boneless, thin-sliced pork chops, not more than ½ inch thick, about 1½ pounds total, trimmed of fat (see Before You Start)

Before You Start It is critical that the pork chops be thin so that they cook through without burning the crumb coating. If you can't find half-inch-thick pork chops, put one-inch-thick chops in the freezer for about 30 minutes to firm them up and then hold them flat on a cutting board with one palm as you cut carefully through the middle with your sharpest knife. This recipe will also work with thinly pounded chicken breasts.

1. ***Make the sauce:*** In a small bowl, whisk the lemon juice with the cumin, coriander, and salt. Whisk the olive oil in slowly, and then stir in the parsley and shallots. Adjust seasoning to taste and set aside.

2. ***Make the pork chops:*** Preheat the oven to 300°F and put an ovenproof serving platter or cookie sheet in the oven to heat up. Put the flour in a wide, rimmed plate or shallow bowl. Whisk the eggs in a similar plate or bowl. Stir together the bread crumbs, coriander, cumin, salt, and a few grinds of pepper in a third similar plate or bowl.

3. In a large sauté pan or skillet set over medium-high heat, heat 2 tablespoons of the olive oil.

4. Pat the pork chops dry, and then dredge them lightly on both sides in the flour, dip them in the egg, and then dip them in the spiced bread crumbs.

5. When the oil is hot, put four of the pork chops in the pan and cook until golden, about 3–4 minutes on each side. As they are cooked, place them in the oven on the warmed platter. Add the remaining 2 tablespoons of olive oil to the pan, and repeat the process with the remaining pork chops.

6. Serve the pork chops drizzled with the parsley sauce.

Pork Loin with Pear and Cornbread Stuffing

This is a classic set of flavors pulled together in a way that is elegant enough for company or for a special holiday meal, but not so difficult you couldn't do it for a nice weekend family supper. We like this easy method of stuffing the pork, which we borrowed from our local butcher in Shelburne. ◇ *Serves: 6–8*

1 center-cut, boneless pork loin roast, about 3½–4 pounds

3 firm but ripe pears, such as Anjou

2 tablespoons unsalted butter

1 shallot, finely minced

1 tablespoon finely chopped fresh sage

1 large, sturdy corn muffin, broken into 1 cup of ¼-inch cubes or rough crumbles (see Before You Start)

¼ cup cider or natural apple juice

1½ teaspoons coarse kosher salt plus more to taste

Freshly ground black pepper to taste

1 tablespoon olive oil

Before You Start It is particularly worth searching out a good piece of meat for this recipe, preferably locally raised and not too lean. You want your pork roast to have a thin layer of fat on top or the meat can dry out. An instant-read thermometer is also critical to judge doneness and prevent overcooking. Allow about 20 minutes per pound to reach 145°F for medium-rare, but start checking the temperature early for best results. You can use one of our Streuseled Maple Corn Muffins (page 260), made without the streusel, for the stuffing.

1. Preheat the oven to 350°F and take the pork roast out of the refrigerator to come to room temperature. Cut the unpeeled flesh of one of the pears into ½-inch cubes.

2. In a large sauté pan or skillet set over medium heat, melt the butter until foamy. Add the cubed pear and shallot and cook, stirring occasionally, until the shallot has softened, 3–4 minutes. Add the sage and corn muffin cubes and cook, stirring occasionally, for another 3–4 minutes. Add the cider, ½ teaspoon of the salt, and a few grinds of pepper. Continue cooking until the cider is absorbed, another 5–7 minutes. Take the stuffing off the heat and cool for 10 minutes until it is easy to handle.

3. Place the pork roast on a cutting board and, with a good sharp knife, cut a deep pocket parallel to the cutting board into the long side of the roast. Start cutting about ¾ inch from the edge and about halfway up from the bottom of the roast, and go almost all the way through the roast to the other side, stopping ¾ inch from the opposite edge.

4. Season the pocket with another ½ teaspoon of the salt and a few grinds of pepper, and fill it with the stuffing. Tie the roast four times around with kitchen twine.

5. Put the roast in a large baking dish or roasting pan with room for the sliced pears around it. Rub the top of the roast with the olive oil and season with the remaining ½ teaspoon of salt and a few grinds of pepper.

6. When you estimate that the roast has about 30 minutes of cooking time left (about 45 minutes in for a 3½-pound roast), slice the remaining two pears into 8 wedges and toss them in the pork roast juices. Spoon some of the juices over the top of the roast. Roast the pork for 15 more minutes, turn the pears, and check the temperature on the pork with an instant-read thermometer.

7. The pears will take another 10–15 minutes to become tender, but depending on its size, your pork roast may be ready. If so, take it out and let it rest, covered loosely with foil, for 10–15 minutes before carving, at which point the pears should be done. Either way, do not skip the rest, which is critical to the roast's juiciness.

8. After the pork has rested, remove the twine and carve it into half-inch-thick slices. Serve stuffed slices of pork topped with the pears and their juices from the roasting pan.

Slow-Roasted Pork Shoulder with Fennel and Orange

[photograph 16]

This dish takes lots of time in the oven, but little time from the cook. It is a bit like pulled pork dressed up for company and is perfect for winter holiday dinners or a cozy après-ski gathering. Maple-Roasted Butternut Squash Puree or Soup (page 202) complements it beautifully. ◇ *Serves: 6–8*

1 large orange, well scrubbed

1 tablespoon whole fennel seeds

1 tablespoon coarse kosher salt

1 teaspoon freshly ground black pepper

3 cloves garlic, minced

1 boneless pork shoulder (Boston butt) roast, 3½–4 pounds, tied (see Before You Start)

1 large fennel bulb (about 1 pound with stalks), trimmed and cut in half lengthwise and then each half crosswise into three pieces

Before You Start If your pork roast comes with a netting to hold it together, cut the netting off and tie the roast a couple of times around with some kitchen twine. There is nothing worse than cutting off the netting after the roast is done and seeing the entire mouthwatering crust go with it. Also, check your label to see if you have bought "enhanced" pork, which is injected with a salty brine. If so, cut the salt in the rub by half.

1. Preheat the oven to 325°F. Zest the orange to yield about 2 teaspoons of finely grated zest, making sure to avoid the bitter white pith. Cut the orange into 8 wedges and set aside.

2. Finely grind the fennel seeds with a mortar and pestle or spice grinder. Then add the salt, pepper, orange zest, and garlic and grind them together into a rough paste.

3. Rub the roast all over with the paste and place in a roasting pan large enough for the roast plus the fennel and orange wedges.

4. Roast the pork for about 3 hours, and then add the fennel and orange wedges, tossing to coat them in the juices. Roast for another 30 minutes and turn the fennel and orange wedges to brown evenly. At about 4–4½ hours' total roasting time, the meat should be completely tender and shred when you pull at it with a fork. The fennel should be soft and caramelized and the orange wedges caramelized.

5. Let the roast sit for a few minutes before carving. Serve with the fennel and orange slices.

Variation Warm any leftover meat, covered, in a low oven alongside corn tortillas. Serve the shredded meat with shredded green cabbage or crisp lettuce and a quick sauce made with sour cream thinned with a little orange juice and seasoned with additional ground cumin, coriander, and salt to taste.

Root-Cellar Vegetables

- ◇ Quick Pickled Carrots and Rutabaga
- ◇ Celery Root Soup with Blue Cheese
- ◇ Beet, Apple, and Radish Salad
- ◇ Cider-Glazed Squash and Arugula Salad
- ◇ Winter Root Slaw
- ◇ Slivered Brussels Sprouts with Bacon and Apple
- ◇ Honey-Glazed Carrots and Turnips
- ◇ Shredded Potato Cake with Leeks and Cheese
- ◇ Roasted Cauliflower with Golden Raisins and Pine Nuts
- ◇ Maple-Roasted Butternut Squash Puree or Soup
- ◇ Golden Flannel Hash

*a*long a curving back road and down a short driveway, you will find a two-acre square of fields anchored by three long greenhouses and a quiet white farmhouse. Vegetable gardens were first planted here at Shelburne Farms over a century ago. At one edge, there are still old brick foundations from the original glass greenhouses, in which gardeners tended exotic palms and cutting flowers, arbors of grapes, and other delicate plants. Today the focus is on more climate-appropriate ingredients for the Inn dining room, and on any given day through late spring, summer, and fall, a small crew of farmers nurtures the harvest, from the first tender peas to knobby stalks of brussels sprouts.

The current Market Garden was established in 1981 by Susan and David Miskell, who moved to Vermont to follow the model of back-to-the-land pioneers Helen and Scott Nearing. After David started his own organic tomato business nearby, Susan continued to run the garden until just a few years ago, meeting each winter to plan with the Inn's chef. "They were also public gardens," she says, explaining that the goal was always more than food. "We spaced the corn four feet apart so the kids could run through it."

Since the Inn is only open seasonally, its menu has never created much demand for storage crops, but the Miskells stockpiled vegetables for themselves, as previous Shelburne Farms gardeners had done to meet Webb family requests for regular deliveries of cabbages, carrots, potatoes, turnips, parsnips, onions, and potatoes through the winter. In the cellar of the farmhouse, the Miskells kept root vegetables bagged in burlap; winter squashes were scattered on shelves throughout the house; onions and garlic hung in the attic.

In winters past, when green vegetables were scarce, Vermonters depended on cabbages and roots from their cellars to make boiled dinners; leftovers became red flannel hash. They scalloped potatoes, turnips, and rutabagas—slicing them thin and drenching them in milk or cream. "Spring-dug" parsnips were left in the ground to be harvested when the ground thawed, sugar-sweet from their chilly hibernation. During the late nineteenth century, Vermont's hardy Green Mountain potato, a now-rare heirloom variety recognized by the Slow Food Ark of Taste, became one of the most popular baking potatoes in the country. Another Vermont heirloom, the sweet and tender Gilfeather turnip (really a rutabaga), is celebrated annually at its own festival.

A Note on Storing Root-Cellar Vegetables
Some general pointers

- If your vegetables come straight from your own garden or a local farm, leave them unwashed if possible, keeping some protective dirt on them. Either way, make sure they are completely dry before storing.
- Check your stored vegetables every few days and remove any that are showing signs of rot, or pull any spoiled leaves off the outside of cabbages.
- Naturally, the longer a vegetable has been out of the ground, the more it uses up its storage reserves. So don't expect a locally grown beet from March to last or taste quite the same as one plucked straight from the earth in October.

Root vegetables such as carrots, celery root, beets, turnips, and rutabagas, as well as leeks, cabbages, and brussels sprouts (best stored on their original stalk if you have room), do best in a cool, dark spot with high moisture to keep them from drying out and wrinkling up. This can range from a wintertime cellar or basement that has a fairly constant temperature of not less than freezing (32°F) and not more than 40°F, to your refrigerator, which will normally run between 35°F and 38°F. If you keep them in a cellar, hold them in plastic buckets, boxes, or bags with some ventilation (wood and humidity are not a great match). To keep humidity high, you may want to splash water regularly on your cellar floors and walls or pack the vegetables in slightly damp sand, as cold-climate gardening guru Eliot Coleman recommends in his book *Four-Season Harvest*. If you're using your refrigerator, simply make sure the vegetable drawer is set to the vegetable option, which is designed to keep moisture in, and cover the vegetables with a damp towel or keep them in a plastic bag with a few holes poked in it.

Potatoes normally do best at the slightly warmer end of the spectrum, between 38°F and 50°F, but since that temperature is hard to find in a modern house, most Vermont farmers recommend keeping them in the refrigerator. The risk is that if they get too cold, their starches can convert into sugar and you could end up with disconcertingly sweet roast potatoes or fries that burn before they cook through. They also need complete darkness to prevent them from turning green, the result of solanine, a natural chemical defense that protects potatoes from predators if they are exposed above ground. Solanine can cause stomach upset, but you can usually peel it off with the skin.

Onions and garlic do best at the same temperature as carrots and turnips (32–35°F) but need to be dry, not moist. The refrigerator or a cool cellar or basement corner is good for them as long as you can keep the humidity level down. An attic may be an option if you have one.

Winter squash also needs a dry spot but does best at higher temperatures (50–55°F). Never refrigerate whole, uncut squash. An attic, basement, or infrequently used guest room where the heat is not always on can be a good choice.

Quick Pickled Carrots and Rutabaga

The refreshing crunch of these pickles is a nice change from roasted, boiled, and pureed root vegetables. Joneve Murphy, the market gardener at Shelburne Farms, is an enthusiastic canner. She would use a fresh cherry bomb pepper from the garden in place of the crushed red pepper. She also goes through the full canning process to keep pickles like these on her cupboard shelves for the whole winter; we went with a quicker refrigerator pickle version, but you could can them if you like. ◇ ***Makes: 2 quarts pickles***

3 large carrots (about ¾ pound), peeled and cut into sticks about 3 inches long by ½ inch wide

1 small rutabaga (about 1 pound), peeled and cut into sticks about 3 inches long by ½ inch wide

1 cup cider vinegar

2 cups water

½ cup sugar

1 tablespoon coarse kosher salt

3 garlic cloves, smashed with the flat side of a knife

1 tablespoon whole fennel seeds

1½ teaspoons whole mustard seeds

¼ teaspoon whole black peppercorns

⅛–¼ teaspoon crushed red pepper to taste

Fresh dill sprigs and fresh fennel fronds (optional)

Before You Start You can do this with just carrots, but the rutabaga adds variety and makes a nice pickle too. You could also use turnips if you like their bite.

1. Prepare a large bowl full of ice water. Bring a medium pot of salted water to a boil over high heat, add the carrots and rutabaga, and boil for 1 minute. Drain immediately and plunge the vegetables into the ice water to stop cooking.

2. In the same pot, combine the cider vinegar, water, sugar, salt, garlic, fennel seeds, mustard seeds, peppercorns, and crushed red pepper. Bring the mixture to a boil and simmer for 3 minutes.

3. Drain the cooled vegetables and put them in a heat-resistant container along with the dill sprigs and fennel fronds, if using. Pour the hot pickling liquid over the vegetables and cool. When they are cool, cover them tightly and refrigerate for at least 12 hours before eating. The pickles can be stored in the refrigerator for about a month.

Celery Root Soup with Blue Cheese

This lovely, simple soup lets the earthy flavor of celery root, also known as celeriac, shine right through. It is the creation of Aaron Josinsky, Rick's sous-chef at the Inn. At the Inn, they add a little butter when pureeing the soup and top each bowl with some roasted apples and a few more crumbles of blue cheese.

◇ *Serves: 4 (can easily be doubled)*

1 medium celery root (celeriac, about 1 pound), peeled and cut into rough 1-inch chunks

3 cups whole or 2 percent milk

½ teaspoon coarse kosher salt plus more to taste

1 cup chicken stock, preferably low sodium

2 ounces crumbled (about ½ cup) best-quality blue cheese, plus more for garnish if desired

1 teaspoon freshly squeezed lemon juice

Before You Start   Don't be scared of celery root's rather gnarly appearance; that's part of its charm and nothing a sharp knife or good vegetable peeler (we like the Y-shaped peelers) can't take care of. Blue cheese lovers may want to add a little more blue, but take care not to overpower the celery root. See page 116 for some of our favorite Vermont blue cheeses.

1. In a medium saucepan, bring the celery root, milk, and salt just to a boil and then reduce the heat to a steady simmer for about 30 minutes until a fork easily pierces a chunk of celery root.

2. Carefully pour the celery root and milk into a blender and blend. (Take care when blending hot liquids—see the Tip on page 14.)

3. Add the chicken stock and blue cheese and blend until completely smooth.

4. Return the soup to the saucepan and warm it gently over medium-low heat. When the soup is hot, take it off the heat and stir in the lemon juice. Adjust seasoning to taste. Serve immediately, sprinkled with additional blue cheese if desired.

Prepare-Ahead Tip: *The soup can be made ahead through step 3 and refrigerated for two or three days. Do not add the lemon juice before reheating because you risk curdling the soup.*

Beet, Apple, and Radish Salad

It seems that the poor beet is always boiled or roasted, so we decided to try it raw and were happy to find a new, refreshing side to it. Resist the urge to toss this all together before serving, because the multicolored layers are really striking.

◇ *Serves: 4*

Buttermilk dressing from Tip, page 25

6 radishes (about 6 ounces), trimmed

1 medium firm, tart, red-skinned apple, such as Empire or Rome, unpeeled (see Before You Start)

1 tablespoon freshly squeezed lemon juice

2 medium beets (about ½ pound total), peeled

2 tablespoons thinly sliced fresh mint leaves

Before You Start   If your apple is particularly juicy, roll the grated shreds in a clean dish towel to remove excess moisture after you've tossed them with the lemon juice. Make sure to grate the beets last or everything will be pink coming out of the grater.

1. Make the Buttermilk Dressing and set aside.

2. Using the medium holes on a box grater or a food processor fitted with the coarse grating blade, grate the radishes and set them aside on a plate. Then grate the apple and toss the shreds in a small bowl with the lemon juice. Lastly, grate the beets.

3. Stir the sliced mint leaves into the prepared dressing. Adjust seasoning to taste.

4. Prepare the salad on individual plates or a communal platter. First arrange a layer of shredded beets, then a layer of apple, and finally radish. Drizzle with the buttermilk dressing and serve immediately.

Living with the Seasons

Joneve Murphy, vegetable farmer,
Shelburne Farms

"It feels really cyclic: you put all your energy into producing the food and you get all of your energy out of it."

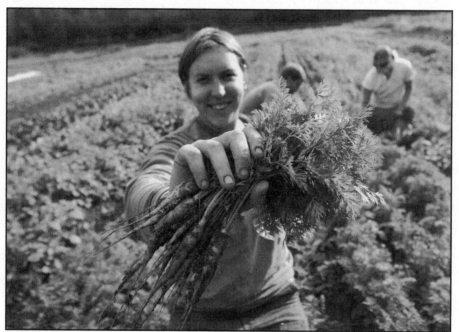

by the beginning of November, the Shelburne Farms season is over and the Market Garden is being put to bed. Twenty-some-odd varieties of tomatoes—bite-size to fist-size; round, oval, teardrop-shaped; crimson, orange, pink, and green with stripes—have come and gone. Tall rows of golden-tasseled sweet corn have reached to the sky and been picked clean. Slender green beans and delicate trays of fragrant baby basil have been painstakingly seeded, tended, and harvested.

And yet the garden still holds treasures. Leeks are there for the harvesting, and rows of crisp carrots and sweet beets are snuggled down beneath the dirt. A plot of hardy greens soldiers on: deep purple, mottled mustard greens; lacinato kale so dark green it's almost black; yellow, red, and purple-spined rainbow chard; green frills of arugula.

Market gardener Joneve Murphy is picking mostly for herself these days, although she invites all Farm employees to help themselves and has already offered up previously harvested, sun-cured winter squash. Today she starts by gleaning baby leeks, which she will slice, sauté with butter and garlic, and freeze. Walking over to grab some mustard greens and broccoli rabe for her lunch, Joneve checks on the garlic she planted earlier in the fall and mulched deeply to protect it until spring. Unseasonably warm weather has her worried, and she does see a few green shoots poking through, but not too many.

Heading back to the house, she pulls a carrot from the ground and rubs it against her pants. "They get really sweet after a frost because all the sugar and energy goes down into their roots," she says, taking a bite. "I've read that if you eat one dirty carrot every day, you get enough B vitamins." The smear from the carrot joins many others on her work pants, a sort of scrapbook of the season gone by, covered with scribbled notes of meeting times mixed in with dirt and splotches of tar from roofing the new garden shed.

This was Joneve's first season at the Farm, her fourth year as a farmer. "I like working hard. I like physical work," she says. "It feels really cyclic: you put all your energy into producing the food, and you get all of your energy out of it . . . I love the seasonality of farming. I think eating seasonally is just healthier. It makes sense." The hardest thing as a farmer, she says, is coping with the weather and learning the nuances of a new piece of land— soils, drainage, patterns of sun and shade. "You just have to know your land," she concludes.

Next year Joneve hopes to set up a root cellar and maybe work with Rick to can some vegetables for the start of the Inn's season. For now, her own freezer and fridge are full and her kitchen shelves lined with pickled green tomatoes, dilly beans, canned beets, and spicy carrots. She is an avid canner, enthusiastically sharing ideas and tips, but not recipes because she never does anything the same way twice. After a long day of work in the fields, she'll come home and cut and bottle and boil and then, as she falls asleep, she says, "You hear the jars go 'plink, plink, plink' as they seal up. It's a good feeling."

Cider-Glazed Squash and Arugula Salad

This salad is modeled after Rick's popular and very pretty Harvest Salad. Since arugula is one of the hardier greens from the Market Garden, it survives early frosts and carries through to the very end of the season. Its bite provides the perfect foil for the dense, sweet cubes of squash. The cider-glazed squash also makes a nice side dish in its own right. ◇ *Serves: 4–6*

1 butternut squash (3 pounds) or pie pumpkin (4 pounds), peeled and seeded, flesh cut into about 20 ¾-inch cubes (see Before You Start)

1 tablespoon olive oil

2 tablespoons apple cider or natural apple juice

½ teaspoon coarse kosher salt

20 raw, peeled hazelnuts

Cider Vinaigrette (page 218)

4 cups (5–6 ounces) baby arugula

½ cup (about 2–3 ounces) crumbled fresh goat cheese

Before You Start   After you've cut your nice, even cubes of squash, you will have some perfectly edible bits left over. See the Variation below for ways to use them.

1. Preheat the oven to 400°F. In a shallow roasting pan or rimmed cookie sheet, toss the squash with the olive oil, apple cider, and salt. Roast the squash for 20–25 minutes, turning once, until it is starting to color and all the liquid has evaporated. Cool the squash.

2. While the squash is roasting, coarsely chop the hazelnuts and put them in the oven in a small baking dish next to the squash to toast for about 10–12 minutes until golden and fragrant. Make the vinaigrette.

3. Arrange the arugula on a platter and toss it with about ⅓ cup of the vinaigrette. Top with the cider-glazed squash cubes, crumbled goat cheese, and toasted hazelnuts and drizzle with a little more vinaigrette as desired.

Variation Try the cider-glazed squash or any leftover squash bits roasted up the same way, tossed with pasta, pearl barley, or wheat berries and some wilted arugula or baby spinach. Top with goat cheese and the toasted hazelnuts.

Prepare-Ahead Tip: *The squash can be roasted up to a day ahead and kept in the refrigerator. Bring to room temperature before serving. The hazelnuts can be toasted ahead and, after cooling, kept sealed at room temperature for a few days.*

Winter Root Slaw

[photograph 13]

In the middle of a Vermont winter, in search of a crisp mouthful of locally grown salad, we created this version of a classic celeri remoulade to add snap to our meals. The sweet crunch of raw parsnip is largely unappreciated, and we know that celery root can be intimidating, but these humble roots are the secret to this salad. It goes well with almost any sautéed or broiled meat or fish. We love it with our Cornmeal Fried Trout with Bacon and Sage (page 153). It's so good that you will miss it in the summer. ◇ **Serves: 4–6**

½ cup crème fraîche (see Before You Start)

2½ tablespoons cider vinegar

1 tablespoon plus 1 teaspoon Dijon mustard

1 teaspoon sugar

1 teaspoon coarse kosher salt plus more to taste

3–4 small parsnips (about ¾ pound), trimmed and peeled

3 medium carrots (about ½ pound), trimmed and peeled

1 small celery root (celeriac, about ¾ pound)

6 scallions, white and light green parts only, thinly sliced

Before You Start   If you can find only large parsnips, buy a little more than 1 pound and cut out and discard the tough inner core. Sour cream can substitute for crème fraîche in this recipe, or you can try making your own (see the Tip on page 73).

1. In a large serving bowl, whisk together the crème fraîche, cider vinegar, mustard, sugar, and salt.

2. Cut the parsnips and carrots into 2-inch matchsticks. Alternatively, run them through a food processor with a coarse grating blade. (Your final slaw will not be quite as crunchy, but it will be just fine.) As you cut or grate them, add the vegetables to the dressing and toss to coat.

3. Using a sharp knife or very good peeler, peel the knobby skin from the celery root and cut or grate per above. Add the celery root to the dressing and toss to coat.

4. Toss in the scallions. Refrigerate for at least 1 hour and up to 2 days. Before serving, adjust seasoning to taste.

Slivered Brussels Sprouts with Bacon and Apple

The greatest enemy to the brussels sprout is cooking; the sprouts are usually varied enough in size that some will overcook while others will be undercooked, and both ends of the spectrum have earned the sprout its generally poor reputation. If you do as we do below and slice them thinly, they will all cook in the same amount of time. ◇ *Serves: 6*

4 slices thick-cut bacon, about ¼ pound

1½ pounds brussels sprouts, stalks trimmed flush, thinly sliced through the root end so that it holds most slices intact

½ teaspoon coarse kosher salt plus more to taste

⅓ cup chicken stock, preferably low sodium

2 teaspoons cider vinegar

2 teaspoons fresh thyme leaves

1 medium firm, tart, red-skinned apple, such as Empire or Rome, unpeeled

Freshly ground black pepper to taste

Before You Start   If you can, try to buy your sprouts still attached to their stalk.

1. In a large sauté pan or skillet, cook the bacon until crisp. Remove the bacon to a plate lined with paper towel. Pour off all but 2 tablespoons of the bacon fat from the pan and discard.

2. Return the pan with the reserved bacon fat to the stove over medium-high heat. Add the brussels sprouts and salt. Cook for 3–4 minutes, stirring, until the sprouts are wilted. Add the chicken stock, cider vinegar, and thyme to the pan and simmer for 3–4 minutes. Taste a sprout to see if it's tender but not mushy.

3. While the sprouts are cooking, cut the apple into matchsticks. When the sprouts are just about done, toss the apple into the hot pan and leave it on the heat for a minute or so. Put the sprouts in a serving bowl, crumble the reserved bacon over them, and adjust seasoning to taste.

Variation   This also works well with a small one-pound cabbage, cored and thinly sliced. If you want the whole dish a little sweeter, replace the chicken stock with apple cider or natural apple juice.

Honey-Glazed Carrots and Turnips

[photograph 12]

This is a classic way to cook carrots to accentuate their natural sweetness. We added turnips for a little variation and for the light bite they bring to the plate. The creamy white turnip wedges also look very pretty against the deep carroty orange.

◇ *Serves: 4–6*

3 large carrots (about ¾ pound), peeled and cut into pieces about 2 inches long by ½ inch wide

3 medium turnips (about ¾ pound), peeled and cut into pieces roughly the same size as the carrots, or about 12 baby turnips, unpeeled and halved with a little green left on top

2 tablespoons honey

2 tablespoons unsalted butter

¾ cup water

½ teaspoon coarse kosher salt plus more to taste

Before You Start You can use just carrots or just turnips. When Rick serves these turnips as a side dish at the Inn, he uses small, sweet Japanese turnips, cut in half with just a hint of the greens on top. They go beautifully with Roast Duck Legs with Sour Cherry Sauce (page 142). You could also substitute rutabagas for turnips if you like. I have found that older stored turnips can develop a fibrous layer under the skin, so investigate as you're peeling and cut that layer off if necessary.

1. In a large skillet or sauté pan that, ideally, fits the carrots and turnips in one layer, put the vegetables, honey, butter, and water. Set the pan over medium-high heat. Bring it to a boil, sprinkle with the salt, and toss to coat the vegetables in the cooking liquid. Reduce the heat to medium and simmer, covered, for about 10 minutes until the carrots are starting to get tender.

2. Remove the cover, toss the vegetables again, and cook uncovered for another 12–14 minutes, tossing occasionally, until the liquid has evaporated to a glaze and the carrots and turnips are tender but not mushy. Adjust seasoning to taste.

Variation If you're doing this with carrots only, try adding 1 teaspoon of coarsely ground toasted cumin seeds—or ½ teaspoon of ground cumin—in step 2.

{ *From the Archives* The Shelburne Farms gardens of the early 1900s grew many varieties of winter storage crops, including Early Jersey Wakefield cabbages, Dalkeith brussels sprouts, the famous Green Mountain potato, and Hubbard squash. A farm report from 1902 recorded an excellent harvest, including 984 bushels of carrots, 620 bushels of turnips, and 610 heads of cabbage.

Shredded Potato Cake with Leeks and Cheese

I used to think you couldn't improve upon the classic potato pancake, until we paired it with some wonderful local cheese and aromatic sautéed leeks for a Vermont twist. This makes a luxurious side dish, or serve full quarter wedges for a main course with a substantial vegetable like Slivered Brussels Sprouts with Bacon and Apple (page 196). ◇ **Serves: 6–8 as a side dish, 4 as a main dish**

¼ cup plus 2 tablespoons olive oil

2 small leeks (about ¾ pound), white and light green parts only, halved lengthwise, thinly sliced, and rinsed thoroughly

1 teaspoon coarse kosher salt plus more to taste

1½ pounds (about 3 large) all-purpose potatoes, such as Green Mountain or Yukon gold, washed but unpeeled

Freshly ground black pepper to taste

¾ cup (about 2–3 ounces) grated Alpine-style cheese, such as Vermont Tarentaise or Gruyère

Before You Start For the crispiest presentation—if you're up for it—flip the potato cake out of the pan onto a serving plate instead of sliding it out so the most recently cooked side is face up.

1. In a 10-inch nonstick sauté pan or skillet, heat 2 tablespoons of the olive oil over medium heat. Reduce the heat to medium-low, add the leeks and ½ teaspoon salt, and cook slowly, stirring occasionally, until soft and golden brown, about 20 minutes. Remove the leeks from the skillet and set aside. Wipe out the skillet with a paper towel to remove any stray pieces of leek.

2. While the leeks are cooking, grate the potatoes using the medium holes of a box grater or the coarse shredding blade of a food processor. Dump the shredded potatoes into a clean dish towel and sprinkle with the remaining ½ teaspoon salt and a few grinds of pepper, tossing with your hands to distribute. Standing over the sink, twist the dish towel around the potatoes to remove as much moisture as possible.

Root-Cellar Vegetables

3. Put the pan back over medium heat with 2 tablespoons of the olive oil. When the oil is shimmering, add half the potato shreds, pressing them firmly into the pan. Top the potato shreds evenly with the leeks and cheese, and then add the remaining potato shreds on top, pressing those firmly into place. Cover the skillet and cook the potato cake until it is golden on the bottom, about 8–10 minutes. (You can peek with a spatula underneath to check every so often.)

4. When the bottom is golden, carefully flip the cake out of the skillet onto a plate. Add the remaining 2 tablespoons of olive oil to the skillet, let it heat up until shimmering, and then slide the potato cake back into the pan. Cook, covered, for another 8–10 minutes until the bottom is golden.

5. Slide the potato cake from the skillet onto a plate. Let sit for 2–3 minutes, cut into wedges, and serve.

Roasted Cauliflower with Golden Raisins and Pine Nuts

If you have never roasted cauliflower, you have missed out. Its nutty taste and slightly crispy texture will make all those memories of waterlogged white blobs vanish right away. We have yet to meet a child who didn't gobble up cauliflower made this way. It's also delicious tossed with a medium-size shaped pasta like ziti or gemelli. ◇ **Serves: 4–6 as a side dish, 4 over pasta as a main course**

1 medium head cauliflower (about 2–3 pounds), cored and broken into bite-size florets

3 tablespoons olive oil

½ teaspoon coarse kosher salt plus more to taste

1 medium leek, white and light green parts only, halved lengthwise, thinly sliced, and rinsed thoroughly

⅓ cup pine nuts

½ cup golden raisins

Freshly ground black pepper to taste

Before You Start You can substitute currants or regular black raisins for the golden raisins, but the result will be a little sweeter.

1. Preheat the oven to 375°F with a rack in the second-highest position. Toss the cauliflower, olive oil, and salt in a shallow roasting pan or rimmed cookie sheet and roast for 15 minutes.

2. Add the leek to the pan and stir. Roast for another 10 minutes.

3. Add the pine nuts to the pan and stir. Roast for another 5 minutes.

4. Remove the pan from the oven, stir in the golden raisins, adjust seasoning as desired, and serve.

Maple-Roasted Butternut Squash Puree or Soup

[photograph 17]

This simple, smooth-as-silk butternut squash puree is a true mouthful of fall. During the dead of winter, its bright golden hue and deep, sweet flavor are most welcome. The puree goes well with many of our main dishes. To turn it into a crowd-pleasing soup, just stir in some stock. Sprinkling the soup with maple-glazed squash seeds (see the variation on Spiced Maple Nuts, page 42) is a nice way to use all edible parts of the squash. ◇ ***Serves: 4–6 as a side dish or soup***

For the puree

1 medium butternut squash (about 3 pounds)

3 tablespoons unsalted butter

3 tablespoons pure maple syrup, Grade B for strongest flavor

1½ teaspoons coarse kosher salt plus more to taste

2 tablespoons crème fraîche (see Before You Start)

For the soup

2–3 cups vegetable or chicken stock, preferably low sodium

1 tablespoon maple syrup whisked into ¼ cup crème fraîche for garnish as desired

Before You Start   If you can't find crème fraîche, substitute heavy cream, which will contribute a similar flavor although not quite the same texture, or try making your own (see the Tip on page 73). The correct amount of salt really brings out the sweetness of the squash in this recipe. Don't be scared; add a little at a time and you'll be amazed at how it rounds out the flavor.

1. Preheat the oven to 350°F. Using a large, sharp knife, cut the squash lengthwise down the middle. Scoop out the seeds and set them aside if you're planning to make maple-glazed seeds. An ice cream scoop or serrated grapefruit spoon works well for this task.

2. Place the squash halves, flesh side up, in a 9 by 13-inch baking dish. Put a tablespoon of butter and a tablespoon of maple syrup in each cavity. Sprinkle each half with ¼ teaspoon of the salt. Cover the pan with foil. Bake for about 1½ hours or until the squash is very soft. Cool just until the squash can be handled.

3. Carefully pour any liquid from the squash cavities into the bowl of a food processor fitted with the metal blade or a blender and then scoop all the flesh into the food processor. Add the remaining tablespoon of butter, remaining tablespoon of maple syrup, remaining teaspoon of salt, and crème fraîche. Puree until completely smooth, stopping to scrape down the sides of the food processor as necessary.

4. If using the dish as a puree, adjust seasoning to taste and serve. (If it's cooled down too much, pop it in the microwave for a minute or so, or back in the oven, covered, for 5–10 minutes.)

5. If making soup, transfer the puree to a medium saucepan, whisk in about 2 cups stock to start, and heat through over medium heat. Thin with additional stock and adjust seasoning to taste. Swirl 1 tablespoon of maple crème fraîche into each bowl of soup and scatter a few maple-glazed squash seeds over the soup as desired.

> **Prepare-Ahead Tip:** *Both the puree and the soup can be made up to a day ahead and kept in the refrigerator. Warm the puree in the microwave or in the oven per step 4 above. Warm the soup gently on the stove, covered.*

Golden Flannel Hash

[photograph 18]

A spin on red flannel hash, the classic country breakfast or light supper, which seems to exist largely in diners nowadays, but deserves more attention. A few old Vermont cookbooks include hash made with potatoes and salt cod; we substituted golden beets for the traditional beets and smoked trout for the corned beef. It makes for a sweet, salty, potatoey, and altogether satisfying dish. Top with a fried egg if you like, and dig in for breakfast, lunch, or supper. ◇ *Serves: 4*

4 medium golden beets (about 1 pound)

3 tablespoons olive oil

3–4 large, waxy potatoes (about 1 pound), such as red or white boiling potatoes

2 tablespoons unsalted butter

1 bunch scallions (8–10 slender scallions), white, light green, and tender dark green parts, sliced ¼ inch thick

6 ounces smoked trout, peeled from the skin and flaked

Coarse kosher salt to taste

Freshly ground black pepper to taste

Before You Start This is an easy recipe, but you do need to allow about 1½ hours to roast and cool the beets and potatoes. They can be cooked up to two days ahead and kept in the refrigerator. Hold off on peeling them until you're ready to finish the dish. Yes, you could make this with red beets, but that would really spoil the whole thing, wouldn't it? Search out golden beets at farmers' markets or well-stocked food markets. You will find smoked trout near the smoked salmon at good fish counters.

1. Preheat the oven to 400°F. Wash and trim the beets and line them up in the center of a long piece of heavy-duty foil. Drizzle with ½ tablespoon of the olive oil. Wrap up the beet package. Wash the potatoes and follow the same directions as for the beets. Put both packages in the oven.

2. Roast the beets and potatoes for 50–60 minutes until a fork easily pierces the largest. (Depending on size, the potatoes are likely to be done first.) Remove from the oven, unwrap, and cool for at least 20 minutes before peeling off the skins and cutting the vegetables into ¼-inch dice.

3. In a large sauté pan or skillet (cast iron is best here), heat the butter and remaining 2 tablespoons of olive oil over medium-high heat. Add the diced potatoes and beets and cook, stirring occasionally, for about 8 minutes until they start to color. Stir in half the sliced scallions and the smoked trout. Cook, stirring occasionally, for another 5–6 minutes until the potatoes and beets are crisp in places, the scallions have wilted, and the trout is warm. Adjust seasoning to taste.

4. Serve topped with a fried egg if desired and scatter with the remaining scallions.

> **Tip:** *If you can find beets with their greens on, buy them, and don't toss the greens even if they're a little limp. They can often be miraculously reinvigorated with a 30-mintue soak in cold water. Wash them well but do not spin dry. Chop coarsely and braise slowly on the stove in a covered pot with just a good pinch of salt, a little chopped onion, and the water left on their leaves. Dress with a squeeze of fresh lemon juice and serve with the hash.*

Root-Cellar Vegetables

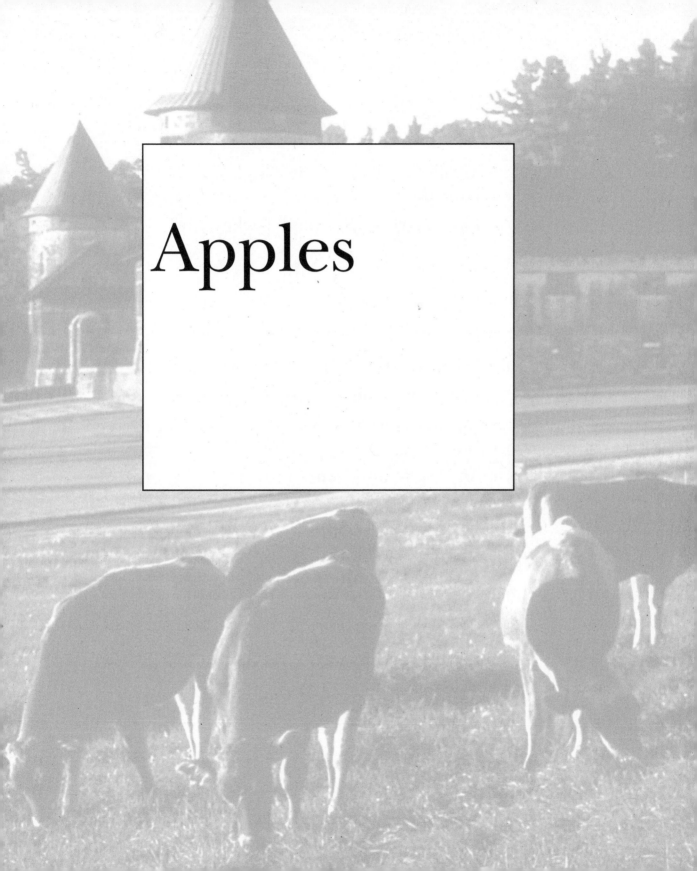

Apples

- Apple and Cinnamon-Sugar Pancakes
- Baked Apple, Smoked Turkey, and Cheddar Strata
- Apple-Rhubarb Chutney
- Cider Vinaigrette
- Honeyed Apple Tea Bread
- Roasted Apple and Plum Parfaits
- Apple-Blackberry Crisp
- Apple-Cranberry Brown Butter Tart
- Apple Pie and Cinnamon Pinwheels
- Oven-Roasted Applesauce and Apple Butter
- Rosemary-Scented Cider Granita

*a*pples have blossomed in Vermont since colonial times, when every hill farmer planted a few trees as part of his homestead. The fruit had many uses; it could be eaten fresh or stored to eat months later; cooked into pies or sauce; dried, canned, or pickled; and made into cider and cider vinegar. Cider—both sweet and hard—was the homegrown beverage of choice and was also sometimes distilled further into applejack or apple brandy. Early apple varieties included Cox's Orange Pippin, brought over from Europe; Fameuse or Snow, known for its snow-white flesh; and the whimsically named Sheep's Nose. There were good keeper apples, apples with the juicy tartness perfect for cider, and naturally sweet apples that collapsed quickly into applesauce.

As apple growing developed into a commercial business in the late 1800s, apple diversity continued, with traveling grafters carrying twigs across the state to ensure the perpetuation of preferred varieties. A few severe winters in the early 1900s, however, devastated many Vermont orchards, and replanting focused on the most disease-resistant, cold-hardy, shippable varieties, led by the now iconic McIntosh. The harvests of the roughly forty commercial apple producers left in Vermont today are still dominated by this shiny red variety, although many are rediscovering some of the older, less familiar apples.

When the Webbs purchased the thirty-seven farms that made up

Shelburne Farms, apple trees were a distinct presence on the land. The location of Shelburne House was, in fact, an apple orchard, and some of the trees were moved to make way for the house. The Webbs continued to cultivate apples and also planted other fruit trees. Varieties included Coe Golden Drop plums, Buerre D'Anjou pears, and Black Tartarian cherries. Apples remained the Farm's major fruit crop, however, and by 1900 there were about six thousand apple trees producing as many as five thousand barrels of fruit annually for family use and for sale. Crews were hired to prune in the spring and to pick in the fall. There were dozens of varieties—from eating apples to cider apples—including Pound Sweets, Russets, Northern Spies, Rhode Island Greenings, Baldwins, Blue Pearmains, Spitzenburgs, and McIntoshes. There are just a few fruit trees left scattered about the property, but place names like Orchard Cove and Cherry Orchard remind us of what was once there.

A Note on Apple Varieties

Asking an apple grower to pick his favorite apple is like asking a parent to pick his favorite child. "It moves with the season," hedges Nick Cowles of Shelburne Orchards, where the roughly five thousand trees encompass around twenty varieties, ranging from old-fashioned and less common Hubbardston Nonesuch, Cox's Orange Pippin, and Rhode Island Greening to lots and lots of McIntosh.

Apples varieties vary, of course, by region; their texture and flavor will also change depending on when they are picked and even on the weather of a certain year. "There are a couple days when Macs are perfect, when their starch is just turning to sugar and they're tart and sweet at the same time. But I don't eat Macs after the end of October," Nick says. "I love Macouns and Cortlands too," he continues. "And the season before last, Galas became my favorite apple for a while. Some years, some apples just really stand out."

That being said, we have noted apple varieties that are well suited to each of the following recipes but since we can't account for all the variables of age, season, and region—or for your tastes—take our recommendations, but experiment with what is available in your own area. And if you see a variety you don't recognize, try something new—especially if it's old.

Apple and Cinnamon-Sugar Pancakes

We fancy the look of these pancakes: a circle within a circle within a circle—and who wouldn't enjoy a little cinnamon-sugar glaze on their pancakes? In fact, one young friend told us they were the only pancakes he'd ever had that tasted good without syrup. (Sorry, sugarmakers.) ◇ ***Makes: about fourteen 3-inch pancakes***

1½ cups all-purpose flour

½ cup whole wheat flour

2 teaspoons baking soda

1 teaspoon baking powder

1 teaspoon table salt

½ teaspoon ground ginger

½ teaspoon ground cinnamon

¼ cup (½ stick) unsalted butter plus more for cooking pancakes

3 tablespoons honey

1 cup plain or vanilla yogurt

1 cup milk

2 large eggs

1 large apple, peeled, cored, and sliced crosswise into very thin circles

Cinnamon sugar made from 3 tablespoons granulated white sugar whisked with 1 teaspoon ground cinnamon

Before You Start Pretty much any apple will work here, although we'd steer clear of those that are supertart and crisp, like Granny Smiths; you want the apple to add a little sweetness and soften up just a bit so it doesn't crunch when you bite into it.

1. In a large bowl, whisk together the all-purpose and whole wheat flours, baking soda, baking powder, salt, ginger, and cinnamon. Set aside. Set a large nonstick griddle or frying pan over medium heat.

2. In a medium bowl in the microwave or a medium saucepan set over medium heat, melt the butter and honey together until they whisk together smoothly. Off the heat, whisk in the yogurt, milk, and eggs. Gently mix the wet ingredients into the dry ingredients just until combined. The batter will be fairly thick.

3. Brush the griddle with a little butter and ladle scant quarter-cupfuls of batter onto the hot griddle, spreading as necessary. Lay an apple slice on the top of each pancake and sprinkle it with a little cinnamon sugar. Cook the pancakes until bubbles form on top and the bottoms are golden brown, about 2–3 minutes.

4. Flip the pancakes and cook for another 2–3 minutes until the second side is golden brown. Serve sprinkled with additional cinnamon sugar and maple syrup as desired.

Baked Apple, Smoked Turkey, and Cheddar Strata

Stratas are savory bread puddings, often with a little less custard and a few more ingredients than the sweet kind. Many are layered with thin slices of bread, but we prefer the craggy texture created by chunks of a good crusty loaf. Sourdough works well here, and if it's a little stale, so much the better. Stratas will happily sit overnight in the refrigerator and then bake in the morning for a perfect brunch dish, or they can be baked and served right away for any meal of the day.

◇ *Serves: 8–10 for brunch, 6–8 for supper*

¾ pound crusty, country-style bread, trimmed of hard crust and cut into 1-inch cubes (about 4–5 cups)

1 tablespoon olive oil

4 large shallots or 1 small onion, thinly sliced (about ⅓ cup)

1 pound smoked turkey (about 2 slices cut about ¾ inch thick), skin discarded, cut into ¾-inch cubes

4 large eggs

1 quart half-and-half

½ teaspoon coarse kosher salt

Freshly ground black pepper to taste

3 medium apples (see Before You Start), peeled, cored, and cut into ½-inch dice

1½ cups (about 6 ounces) coarsely grated sharp cheddar

Before You Start   For this dish you want a semitart, crisp apple that is not so juicy that it leaches lots of liquid nor so soft that it completely disappears into the custardy bread. Flavor-wise, it should stand up to the smoked meat and rich cheddar. Try Granny Smith, Macoun, Empire, Winesap, or Cox's Orange Pippin if you're lucky enough to find it.

1. Preheat the oven to 375°F. Lightly oil a 9 by 13-inch baking dish. Lay the bread on a cookie sheet and toast it in the oven for 10 minutes, then set aside to cool. Reduce the oven temperature to 350°F.

2. In a large sauté pan or skillet set over medium-high heat, heat the olive oil. Add the shallots and cook, stirring occasionally, until softened, 3–4 minutes. Add the turkey to the pan and cook, turning occasionally, until lightly browned, 5–7 minutes. In a medium bowl, whisk together the eggs, half-and-half, salt, and a few grinds of pepper.

3. In the prepared baking dish, evenly distribute half the shallot-turkey mixture, half the apple, and half the cheese, making one layer. Top with all the bread, then the remaining shallot-turkey mixture and apple in a third layer. Pour the egg mixture over it all and push the bread down to submerge it in the custard. Sprinkle the remaining cheddar over the top.

4. Bake for 45–50 minutes until the top is golden brown and the custard is set. Let stand for 5 minutes before serving.

Prepare-Ahead Tip: *The strata can be prepared through step 3, covered with lightly greased foil and refrigerated overnight. Allow 15 minutes of additional baking time, and keep it covered with foil for the first 25 minutes in the oven.*

Apple-Rhubarb Chutney

[photograph 3]

*This versatile sweet-tart condiment can go many ways. As originally created with a touch of cider vinegar, it is a savory complement to grilled or roasted pork, ham, or roast chicken. It also works as a lighter Vermont version of the Branston Pickle chutney traditionally served with a ploughman's lunch, and is also perfect for a cheese plate. If you omit the cider vinegar, you will have a gently tart compote to spoon over vanilla ice cream, stir with yogurt, or serve with our Maple–Cream Cheese Pound Cake (page 242). ◇ **Makes: about 2½ cups chutney**

½ cup apple cider or natural apple juice

½ cup pure maple syrup, Grade B for strongest flavor

2 tablespoons cider vinegar

1 sprig fresh rosemary

2 medium apples (see Before You Start), peeled, cored, and cut into ½-inch cubes

½ pound fresh or frozen rhubarb sliced ½ inch thick (about 2 cups)

½ cup dried sweetened tart cherries

Before You Start   Apples in this chutney should hold their shape and can be fairly sweet, as the rhubarb more than delivers on the tart quotient. Try Braeburn, Empire, Fuji, Northern Spy, Paula Red, or Winesap. When rhubarb starts popping up in May in Vermont, even long-keeping local apples are pretty much done. Rhubarb, however, will produce all season long if you keep cutting it and the weather doesn't turn scorching. In fact, the thicker later-season stalks work especially well in this recipe. Frozen rhubarb will also work fine; you just may need to simmer the chutney a little longer. If you can't find rhubarb, use a total of one cup of dried sweetened tart cherries instead.

1. In a medium saucepan set over medium-high heat, combine the cider, maple syrup, cider vinegar, and rosemary. Bring to a simmer and cook for 5 minutes.

2. Carefully remove the rosemary sprig and discard. Stir in the apple, rhubarb, and cherries. Simmer for another 5–7 minutes until the fruit is just tender but not mushy. Cool and store in a clean jar in the refrigerator for up to two weeks.

Finding the Sweet Spot
Nick Cowles, apple grower,
Shelburne Orchards

"I love my relationship with my community through the orchard, that people come out and I get to grow something people love."

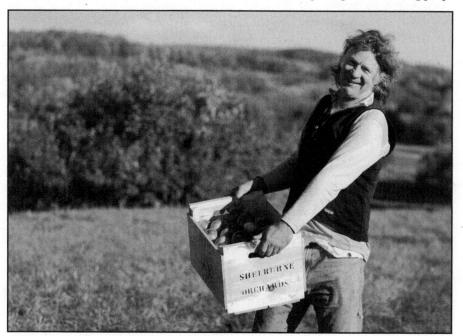

ick Cowles turns the spigot on a small wooden cask, and an eye-smarting, fruity whiff flows out along with a steady trickle of apple cider vinegar. He takes a swallow and smiles broadly. "I have a spoonful every day," he says. "I love it because it's old-fashioned and because it's from the earth."

Emerging from the kitchen into bright fall sunshine, Nick blinks. It's mid-September, and Shelburne Orchards is at its busiest. The crew is cleaning up from last weekend's small farms festival and preparing for the pie festival that comes next. A couple of times a week, busloads of schoolchildren arrive to learn about the life of an apple orchard. There are pies to bake, cider doughnuts to make, apples to pick and pack or press—not to mention orders to take and deliver. Even the crickets chirping among the trees sound busy.

The small store set up on a porch in front of the Shelburne Orchards packing house is piled high with pale freckled Ginger Golds, mottled red and green Gravensteins, and the first of the ubiquitous McIntosh. There are even buckets of small, blushing peaches from trees that have borne fruit for the first time in three years thanks to a warm winter. A local pulls in to pick up an order, and a couple from out of state wants to pick their own. Nick dispatches a young helper to help them navigate their way among the rows of apple trees that flow down the hill toward a glittering Lake Champlain. Above the water, the Adirondacks cut crisply into an intense blue sky.

Nick grew up on the sixty-acre, century-old orchard a couple of miles south of Shelburne Farms, to whom he now sells apples. In the 1970s he became the first in his family to try to make a full-time living off of the orchard. "It was always a hobby for my dad," he says, "but he loved it, too. My best times with him were in the orchard, him teaching me how to graft. I first understood it and fell in love with it through him."

"When I took over, I was young and optimistic," he continues. "I thought I was going to turn the whole orchard organic." It was a struggle, he recalls, outlining the challenges of growing apples organically in Vermont's climate. "I couldn't make my payments. I got angrier and angrier. I almost lost the whole place." He takes a deep breath. "Then I reestablished what was most important: If I sold, everybody loses out." Nick allowed himself to start using low-spray pest management practices, and he slowly got back on his feet and built up the business. He still devotes ten acres to organic practices, but they have had only minimal success.

Although September and October bring the most people to Shelburne Orchards, spring—when everything is starting to wake up from its deep winter slumber—is also a busy time for an apple farmer. Nick spends time pruning and checking how the trees fared through the cold, and in May he celebrates the new season with a supper under the blossoms. "I love my relationship with my community through the orchard," he says, "that people come out and I get to grow something people love. The rest of the year I love the quiet."

Cider Vinaigrette

This vinaigrette features two of Vermont's signature flavors and graces many fall salads at the Inn, including the Cider-Glazed Squash and Arugula Salad (page 194). Rick also uses it with another wonderful combination: arugula with thinly sliced Shelburne Orchards Cortland apples (they and Empires would both work well because they don't turn brown as soon as they are cut), Spiced Maple Nuts (page 41), and thin shavings of Shelburne Farms' prized clothbound cheddar. Or try the dressing over baby spinach leaves, golden raisins, toasted slivered almonds, and a little fresh goat cheese. ◇ ***Makes: 1 cup***

½ cup apple cider or natural apple juice

2 tablespoons cider vinegar

1 teaspoon pure maple syrup, Grade B for strongest flavor

1 shallot, finely minced

½ teaspoon coarse kosher salt plus more to taste

¼ cup olive oil

Freshly ground black pepper to taste

Before You Start   When Rick makes this dressing at the Inn, he reduces the apple cider slowly on the stove by about half to intensify it; you're welcome to do that, but we like it just fine without that time-consuming step.

1. In a blender or mini food processor, blend together the cider, cider vinegar, maple syrup, shallot, and salt.

2. Gradually add the olive oil and blend to emulsify. Adjust seasoning to taste.

From the Archives The correspondence of Edward Gebhardt, longtime manager of Shelburne Farms for Lila and Seward Webb, mentions apples frequently because they took much effort to maintain, harvest, store, sell, and ship to the Webbs, their friends and family, and various wholesalers. He noted that apples were being pressed into cider, identified Pound Sweets as "good eating apples," and specifically reported that the fruit of one orchard was being used for applesauce.

Honeyed Apple Tea Bread

Relatively few people realize that apple orchards still depend on a very small but busy guest worker to ensure a good harvest: the honeybee. Every commercial Vermont orchard brings in hives of honeybees for the blossom season. Other insects and even some birds and bats can pollinate, but none are as industrious. "They just don't get out and do it like the honeybee," confirms Nick of Shelburne Orchards. It seemed appropriate for that reason to pair the two in this very light, honey-scented tea bread, perfect for brunch, tea, or a blossom season picnic in an apple orchard. ◇ **Makes: one 9 by 5-inch loaf**

For the tea bread

2 cups all-purpose flour

2 teaspoons baking powder

½ teaspoon table salt

4 large eggs

¼ cup honey

¾ cup granulated white sugar

½ cup (1 stick) unsalted butter, melted

1 tablespoon apple brandy, such as Calvados (optional)

2 medium apples, peeled, cored, and cut into ¼-inch dice (about 2 cups; see Before You Start)

1 tablespoon finely grated lemon zest

For the glaze

¼ cup confectioner's sugar

3 tablespoons honey

2 tablespoons freshly squeezed lemon juice (from the same lemon used for zest)

Before You Start   Use a nice sweet apple that will hold its shape when baked, such as Ginger Gold or Golden Delicious. Zest the lemon first, then cut it in half to juice it.

1. Preheat the oven to 350°F. Generously butter a 9 by 5-inch loaf pan. In a medium bowl, whisk together the flour, baking powder, and salt.

2. In the bowl of a standing mixer fitted with the whisk attachment, or using a handheld electric mixer, beat the eggs on high speed with the honey and white sugar until light, about 8–10 minutes. Using a spatula, gently fold the flour mixture into the egg mixture alternately with the melted butter.

3. Stir in the apple brandy, if using, and then the diced apple and lemon zest. Mix just to combine and make sure there are no flour pockets, but do not overmix. Spread the batter into the prepared pan.

4. Bake for 45–50 minutes until the top is golden brown and a cake tester or toothpick comes out clean. If the top gets too dark, cover it with foil. Cool the tea bread in its pan on a rack for about 5 minutes, then remove it from the pan and place it on a serving platter to glaze while still warm.

5. While the tea bread is cooling, prepare the glaze. Measure the confectioner's sugar into a small bowl and whisk it to remove lumps. In a small saucepan over medium-low heat or in a small bowl in your microwave, warm the honey with the lemon juice for about 1 minute and whisk them together. Whisk the warm honey mixture into the confectioner's sugar until smooth and pour it immediately over the warm tea bread. Cool before serving.

> **Tip:** If you prefer a tea bread with a flat top and no crown, when the top is just starting to set—about 20 minutes into baking—use a sharp knife to cut a ½-inch-deep slit down the middle of the cake lengthwise.

Roasted Apple and Plum Parfaits

[photograph 19]

Just like the Webbs originally at Shelburne Farms, quite a few Vermont apple orchards have a few plum trees, some of which bear fruit late in the summer and deliver sweet, soft plums to pair beautifully with tart, crisp, early-season apples. This simple but elegant dessert combines deep maple-caramel flavors, crunch, and cream all in one to create a sophisticated—but not overly so—older cousin of a crisp. ◇ **Serves: 6–8**

6 large apples (about 2½ pounds; see Before You Start), peeled, cored, and cut into ½-inch dice or ⅛-inch half-moons

8 large red or black plums (about 2 pounds), halved, pitted, and each cut into 8 half-moons

4 tablespoons unsalted butter, cut into ¼-inch cubes

1 teaspoon cinnamon

½ cup pure maple syrup, Grade B for strongest flavor

1 pint heavy cream

Sugar to sweeten whipped cream (optional)

Maple-Almond Brittle (page 270)

Before You Start   You'll want an apple with a little bite and some firmness to complement the sweet plums. Try Northern Spy, Rhode Island Greening, Macoun, or Empire. Each part can be prepared ahead and the dessert assembled right before serving. If the roasted fruit has been refrigerated, make sure to bring it to room temperature before putting the parfaits together.

1. Preheat the oven to 375°F. In a large roasting pan or rimmed cookie sheet, toss together the fruit, butter, cinnamon, and maple syrup.

2. Roast for 30–35 minutes, stirring once or twice, until the fruit is tender and caramelized but not completely mushy. (The juices will be released and some will evaporate.)

3. While the fruit is roasting, whip the cream (with a little sugar if desired).

4. To serve, either spoon fruit into bowls and top with whipped cream and Maple-Almond Brittle or, for a more elegant presentation, dig out grandma's parfait glasses and layer fruit, whipped cream, and crunch and repeat, topping with a decorative shard of brittle.

Variation Roasted fruit is a wonderful thing. Be inspired by what is seasonal and available in your local market. Just use roughly the same quantities of two complementary fruits, such as pears and plums, peaches or apricots and sweet cherries, or apples and figs. Softer fruits will take less time to roast, so check them at 20 minutes.

Tip: *Cream whips up faster if you pop the bowl and beaters in the freezer for as little as 15 minutes before using.*

Apple-Blackberry Crisp

Even though it's really a simple, homey dish, when apple crisp made with Shelburne Orchards' fruit is on the Inn's dessert menu in the fall, it outsells everything else by far. They make it in individual oval ramekins and lay the rich, crunchy topping on thick, which seems to make everyone very happy. ◇ ***Serves: 8–10***

For the topping

1 cup packed light brown sugar

¾ cup packed dark brown sugar

1¼ cups all-purpose flour

2 teaspoons ground cinnamon

¼ teaspoon ground nutmeg

¼ teaspoon table salt

¾ cup (1½ sticks) unsalted butter, cold, cut into ¼-inch cubes

½ cup old-fashioned oats (quick-cooking are fine, but not instant)

For the filling

3 pounds apples (about 9 medium), peeled, cored, and thinly sliced (see Before You Start)

3 cups fresh or frozen unthawed blackberries

⅓ loosely packed cup light brown sugar

2 tablespoons all-purpose flour

1 teaspoon ground cinnamon

Before You Start   We added blackberries for something a little different, but of course you can make a purist version with just apples. Give yourself one additional pound of apples (about three more). The choice of apples here is very much up to you. If you like your crisp filling to be sweet and saucy, go for McIntosh or Fuji. If you like a little tartness and want to keep some texture, pick Jonathan, Paula Red, or Ida Red.

1. Preheat the oven to 350°F.

2. Prepare the topping: Using a food processor, pulse the light and dark brown sugars, flour, cinnamon, nutmeg, and salt together to combine. Add the butter and oatmeal and pulse just until the topping is gravelly with pieces of oatmeal still visible. Set aside.

3. Prepare the filling: In a 9 by 13-inch baking pan or other shallow 3½–4 quart baking dish, toss together the apples, blackberries, sugar, flour, and cinnamon. Cover generously with the topping, using your hands to squeeze together handfuls and pat them into place.

4. Bake for 45–50 minutes until the topping is dark golden brown and the apples are soft.

Variation   Other great apple crisp combinations include apple with fresh or frozen sour cherries or cranberries (double the sugar in both cases), and apple with plums or pears. If you're lucky enough to live in peach or apricot country, those also work beautifully in this recipe. Double the flour in the filling and shave 10–15 minutes from the baking time.

Apple-Cranberry Brown Butter Tart

For an elegant end to a holiday or other special fall or winter meal, the combination of apples and cranberries against a backdrop of sweet, nutty, brown butter is truly special and very pretty too. ◇ ***Makes: one 10-inch tart***

For the crust

1¼ cup all-purpose flour

½ teaspoon table salt

¼ cup granulated white sugar

½ cup (1 stick) unsalted butter, cold, cut into ¼-inch cubes

1 large egg yolk

1–2 tablespoons ice water

For the filling

½ cup (1 stick) unsalted butter

2 large eggs

⅓ cup packed light brown sugar

⅓ cup plus 2 teaspoons granulated white sugar

¼ cup all-purpose flour

Pinch table salt

1 cup (about 4 ounces) fresh or frozen unthawed cranberries

2 medium apples (see Before You Start)

To finish

3 tablespoons apple jelly, melted

Before You Start   Choose apples that will hold their shape when thinly sliced and add a sweet note to the tart cranberries. Cortland, Empire, and Rome have all worked well for us. Golden Delicious would also be a fine choice.

1. Preheat the oven to 400°F with a rack in the lowest position.

2. *Prepare the crust:* Combine the flour, salt, and sugar in the bowl of a food processor and pulse to combine. Add the butter and pulse until the mixture looks like cornmeal, about fifteen 1-second pulses. In a small bowl or cup, whisk together the egg yolk and 1 tablespoon of the ice water. Drizzle the egg yolk mixture through the food processor's feed tube and pulse about fifteen times, just until the dough forms large lumps. You may need to add the second tablespoon of ice water.

3. Dump the dough out into a 10-inch tart pan, ideally with a removable bottom. Starting with the sides, press the dough lightly with your fingers to make a ¼-inch-thick crust. Distribute the remaining dough evenly over the bottom of the pan and cover it with a piece of plastic wrap. Pat the dough into place with your fingers or use the rounded bottom of a measuring cup to even it out. Remove the plastic wrap and prick the crust about a dozen times with a fork. Bake the crust for 15–17 minutes or until the edge is golden brown and the center is golden. Remove the crust to a cooling rack. Reduce the oven temperature to 350°F.

4. *While the crust is baking, prepare the filling:* In a small, light-colored saucepan set over medium heat, melt the butter and cook until light brown solids appear on the bottom of the pan, about 7–8 minutes. Watch closely toward the end, and when you see brown appear in the butter, take the pan off the heat immediately.

5. In the bowl of a standing mixer fitted with the paddle attachment, beat the eggs with the brown sugar and ⅓ cup of the white sugar at high speed until thick, about 3–4 minutes. Beat in the flour and salt and then the browned butter, including the light brown solids. Coarsely chop ¾ cup of the cranberries and stir them into the brown butter batter. (You can chop the cranberries in the food processor used for the crust. Just wipe it out with a paper towel.)

6. Peel the apples and cut them into quarters. Cut out the core with a paring knife and slice each quarter into about 6–8 thin half-moons.

7. Spread the brown butter and cranberry batter evenly into the bottom of the tart shell. Then arrange two circles of overlapping apple slices around the outside edge of the tart, leaving a 2-inch open circle in the middle.

8. Arrange the remaining ¼ cup of cranberries in the open circle, pressing them down a little into the batter. Sprinkle them with the remaining 2 teaspoons of sugar.

9. Bake the tart for 40–45 minutes until the filling is light golden brown and the apples golden. Cool the tart on a rack for about 1 hour and then brush the apples with the melted apple jelly. Let sit 10 minutes before serving.

Apple Pie and Cinnamon Pinwheels

[*photograph* 20]

Apple pie warms the heart, but failed piecrusts have caused many a heartache, so we've fine-tuned this crust recipe to ensure success for even the least experienced baker. The truth of the matter is that practice makes perfect, and if you can find a great pie baker to learn from, you'll have a big advantage. Many Vermonters have told me of the cinnamon pinwheel cookies their mothers or grandmothers would rustle up out of the scraps left from rolling out pie dough. A perfect—and tasty—example of putting everything to good use. ◇ Makes: one 10-inch (or 9-inch, preferably deep-dish) pie plus fifteen to twenty 1-inch cinnamon pinwheels

For the crust

½ cup milk

3 cups all-purpose flour plus more for rolling

2 tablespoons granulated white sugar

½ teaspoon table salt

6 tablespoons vegetable shortening, cold

1 cup (2 sticks) unsalted butter, cold, cut into ¼-inch cubes

For the filling

3 pounds (about 6–8 large) apples

¾–1 cup packed light brown sugar

1 teaspoon cinnamon

2–3 tablespoons all-purpose flour

¼ teaspoon table salt

2 tablespoons unsalted butter, sliced into thin pats

To finish

Milk to brush crust

Granulated white sugar to sprinkle over crust

Before You Start   A thrifty Vermont farmwife would have used lard for her crusts or gone for the purist butter version, but since good lard is hard to find nowadays and achieving a tender, all-butter crust can be challenging, we've compromised with a combination of butter for flavor and vegetable shortening for texture and ease, plus milk to heighten the sweet dairy flavor. A food processor—while not traditional—is the easiest way to pull together a tender crust. If you don't have a food processor, cut the fats into the flour with two forks or a pastry blender to reach the described texture, and then stir in the milk. If you are concerned about your pie bubbling over, put a foil-covered cookie sheet on the bottom rack in the oven under the rack you start the pie on, but be forewarned that it may take longer for your bottom crust to bake. I strongly recommend a glass pie pan because you can actually check the bottom crust.

As far as apples go, there are many schools of thought. An old Vermont saying goes, "A Spy in your pie," and many old-timers still search out Northern Spies. Some people use a mix to balance the flavor. Cortland, Empire, Fuji, Baldwin, and Ida Red all work well, and while Golden Delicious may be too sweet for some, they hold their shape very well. On the flip side, we find Granny Smiths too tart, but others like them.

1. Prepare the crust: Place the milk in the freezer to chill. In the bowl of a food processor, pulse together the flour, sugar, and salt to blend. Cut the shortening into six pieces and pulse it into the flour mixture with about six 1-second pulses until the mixture forms even crumbs. Add the butter and blend it into the flour mixture with about ten 1-second pulses until the mixture is pebbly with a few bigger pea-size lumps of butter.

2. Pour ¼ cup of the chilled milk into the feed tube and pulse three or four times. Continue to add the milk by the tablespoonful, pulsing two or three times after each addition, until large chunks of dough come together. (You will probably use all the milk unless it's quite humid out.)

3. Get out two plastic bags or cut two square pieces of plastic wrap before your hands get all doughy in the next step. Turn the dough into a large bowl and gather it together into two equal balls. (You should still be able to see some small lumps of butter in the dough.) Flatten the balls lightly into disks and put them in the bags or wrap them up. Refrigerate the dough for about 30 minutes.

4. Preheat the oven to 425°F with two racks set in the lowest and the second-lowest slots.

5. While the pie dough is chilling, prepare the filling: Peel and slice the apples into ⅛-inch-thick slices (you should have about 8 cups of fruit) and toss them with ¾ cup of the brown sugar, the cinnamon, 2 tablespoons of the flour, and the salt in the bowl you used for the dough. If your apples seem very juicy, add another tablespoon of flour. If they are quite tart, add a little more brown sugar.

6. Unwrap one chilled ball of dough and place it on a lightly floured surface. With a lightly floured rolling pin, roll the ball from the center out until you have a circle about ⅓ inch thick and about 13 inches in diameter. (You may need to patch a little as you roll.) Gently slide a metal spatula under the rolled-out crust, fold it over the rolling pin, and transfer it to your pie pan. Fit the dough to the pan, patching as necessary, and fill it with the apples, mounding them toward the center. Top the apples with the pats of butter.

7. Roll out the second ball of dough in the same way as the first. Brush the edge of the bottom crust with water. Transfer the top crust to the pie using a spatula and rolling pin as before. Leaving a ¼-inch overhang all around, trim the excess with a sharp knife or scissors. Seal and crimp the edges.

8. Brush the top lightly with milk, cut four or five generous vents, and sprinkle with sugar. Set the pie in the oven on the rack in the second-lowest slot and bake for 25 minutes.

9. Lower the oven temperature to 350°F and move the pie to the lowest rack. If the crust edge is already well browned at this point, which it often is, use a long, thin piece of foil to cover and protect just the edge of the crust. Bake for another 25–30 minutes, or until the top crust is golden brown, the apples give when poked through one of the vents, and the bottom crust is golden (it never gets quite as dark as the top).

10. ***When the pie goes in the oven, make the cinnamon pinwheels:*** Roll any extra pie dough into a rough rectangle about ¼ inch thick, sprinkle with a little cinnamon and sugar, roll like a jelly roll, and then slice into ¼-inch-thick rounds. Bake the pinwheels on an ungreased cookie sheet in the oven above the pie, and they'll be golden in about 8–10 minutes.

Tip: *If you have time and freezer space, it helps to pop the unbaked pie in the freezer for 30 minutes or so before baking. The chill will help the crust set before the apples shrink and give you a nicely domed crust.*

Oven-Roasted Applesauce and Apple Butter

The aroma that seeps into every nook and cranny of your house is reason alone to make applesauce. Apple butter is just sauce taken a few steps further into a wonderfully intense spread. I love this recipe because the oven does most of the work and as long as you have a food mill, you don't need to peel the apples. In fact, depending on their color, the skins can give your sauce a beautiful rosy hue (apple butter will end up a deep, rich brown no matter what). Applesauce and apple butter have so many uses I hardly know where to start. Try them as a side to pork dishes such as our Ale-Braised Kielbasa with Sauerkraut (page 175), as a condiment for a cheese plate, rolled in crepes and topped with Maple-Butterscotch Sauce (page 271), or swirled with yogurt and layered with Maple-Nut Granola (page 258) for a breakfast or dessert parfait. ◇ **Makes: about 7 cups of applesauce or 1¼ cups of apple butter (or you can double the quantity, use two roasting pans, and then consolidate into one at the apple butter stage)**

5 pounds apples, about 15 medium (see Before You Start), cored and cut into 8 wedges each, peeled unless you have a food mill

½ cup apple cider or natural apple juice

¼–½ cup maple syrup depending on tartness of apples, Grade B for strongest flavor

4 whole cinnamon sticks

4 whole star anise, divided and tied up in 2 cheesecloth bundles

Before You Start I strongly recommend buying a food mill; the sturdy plastic versions are not pricey and will earn back their cost in no time just between making applesauce and making fluffy mashed potatoes. If you don't have a food mill, you will need to peel the apples first. Nick of Shelburne Orchards likes using Paula Reds for a soft pink sauce. Another local apple grower recommends a mix of Cortland, Macoun, Spartan, and Liberty for a nicely balanced sauce. I usually take some applesauce out after 30 minutes of oven time and continue making the rest into apple butter.

1. Preheat oven to 375°F. In a large, heavy, shallow roasting pan, toss the apples with the cider and maple syrup. Distribute the cinnamon sticks and star anise. Roast until the apples are very soft, about 30–45 minutes depending on apple variety.

2. Pull out the cinnamon sticks and star anise and set them aside if you are planning to make apple butter. Run the apples through a food mill or, if they were peeled, mash them roughly with a potato masher or puree them in a food processor or blender. You're now done if you wanted applesauce.

3. For apple butter, reduce the oven temperature to 300°F and spread the applesauce back into the roasting pan with the reserved cinnamon sticks and star anise. Taste and stir in more maple syrup if desired.

4. Bake until a dollop of the apple mixture on a plate releases no liquid, usually 1–1½ hours, but this can vary depending on your apples. (If you had significantly less than 7 cups of sauce at step 3, you can expect it to go faster.) Stir every 30 minutes, taking particular care to move the sauce away from the sides of the pan. You will want to do this more frequently the longer you cook it.

5. Remove the cinnamon sticks and star anise and cool before storing in the refrigerator. Apple butter or applesauce will keep up to two weeks in the refrigerator or can be frozen for several months.

Variation Try the same basic technique with apples plus some pears or plums. Apricots and peaches with apples are also a lovely combination. A friend of mine always throws a cup or two of cranberries in her applesauce for a bright pink hue. The spices, of course, can be customized to taste. Some people love ginger, others cardamom—both of which are best added ground rather than whole like the cinnamon and star anise.

Rosemary-Scented Cider Granita

This icy, crunchy, frozen dessert tastes like a walk in a Vermont apple orchard with a breeze wafting in from a nearby evergreen forest. It was inspired by a surprisingly refreshing Douglas fir sorbet I had some years ago at the Herbfarm Restaurant in Washington State. For a more elaborate version of Vermont sugar on snow, you could serve it topped with warm Maple-Butterscotch Sauce (page 271)

◇ *Makes: 1 quart*

4 cups apple cider

1 sprig fresh rosemary, 4 inches, or two 2-inch sprigs

1. Pour the cider into a bowl and pull the rosemary leaves from the stalk into the bowl, bruising them with your fingers as you do so. Add the rosemary stem and let the cider steep for 1 hour at room temperature.

2. Pour the cider through a sieve into a shallow metal container such as a 9 by 13-inch baking dish or a roasting pan. Place it carefully in your freezer.

3. Freeze for about 2 hours, mixing with a fork to break up ice crystals every 30 minutes or so until it is all frozen flakes.

Prepare-Ahead Tip: *The granita can be made ahead and kept in the original metal container, covered, in the freezer for up to a week. Just scrape it up again if it becomes too solid.*

Sweet
Milk

- ◇ Orange-Yogurt Coffee Cake
- ◇ Cream Scones with Golden Raisins
- ◇ Maple–Cream Cheese Pound Cake
- ◇ Hot Milk Sponge Cake
- ◇ Chocolate–Sour Cream Cake with Bittersweet Chocolate Frosting
- ◇ Cup Custards with Pears Poached in Sweet Wine
- ◇ Sour Cherry–Chocolate Cheesecakes
- ◇ Fresh Mint Ice Cream
- ◇ Buttermilk-Plum Sherbet

*f*or close to two centuries, Vermont has been a dairy state where fresh milk, cream, and butter usually traveled only a few miles from the cow to the kitchen—and more often it was just a barn's throw between the two. Desserts and pastries would be sadly bereft without butter, of course, but there are also the sweet rewards of light, tangy yogurt; rich cream, cream cheese, and sour cream; the refreshing acidity of buttermilk; and even just plain old milk.

Thick fresh cream was poured over fruit cobblers and crisps and their fancifully named cousins: buckles, grunts, slumps, and pandowdies. Along with farm-raised eggs, cream or rich milk was also the foundation of many a soft, smooth pudding or custard.

Old Vermont cookbooks often specify rich milk—milk used before the cream rose and was poured off—or sweet milk, as distinguished from soured, which the thrifty farmwife also put to good use in tender pancakes, doughnuts, cakes, and cookies. She would surely laugh at modern cooks' buying buttermilk in a carton from the supermarket.

Orange-Yogurt Coffee Cake

This is a very pretty breakfast, brunch, or tea cake, infused with orange and tender with yogurt. It was created by Christine Frost, a former pastry chef for the Inn, and is especially good glazed with Side Hill Farm's apricot-orange marmalade, an Inn breakfast-time favorite. ◇ **Makes: 1 large Bundt or tube cake**

For the cake

2 large oranges, washed well

2 cups all-purpose flour

1½ teaspoons baking powder

½ teaspoon baking soda

1 teaspoon table salt

6 tablespoons unsalted butter, at room temperature

1 cup granulated white sugar

2 large eggs

¾ cup vanilla or plain yogurt, not nonfat

1 teaspoon pure vanilla extract

For the glaze

2 tablespoons unsalted butter

2 tablespoons freshly squeezed orange juice from oranges above

½ cup apricot-orange marmalade or orange marmalade

1 teaspoon confectioner's sugar (optional)

Before You Start   Side Hill Farm marmalade can be bought through Shelburne Farms (see Sources, page 273).

1. **Make the cake:** Preheat the oven to 350°F. Zest both oranges to yield about 1 tablespoon of finely grated orange zest, making sure to avoid the bitter white pith. Squeeze the oranges to yield ½ cup plus 2 tablespoons of juice. Set the zest and juice aside.

2. Prepare a large (10–12 cup) Bundt or tube pan by buttering it very well, dusting it with flour, and putting it in the refrigerator. In a medium bowl, whisk together the flour, baking powder, baking soda, and salt.

3. In the bowl of a standing mixer fitted with the paddle attachment or with a handheld electric mixer, cream the butter and sugar together until light and fluffy, about 5 minutes. Add the eggs one at a time, beating until fully incorporated.

4. In a small bowl, whisk together the reserved orange zest, ½ cup of the reserved orange juice, the yogurt, and the vanilla. With the standing mixer on low speed, add the dry ingredients and wet ingredients to the creamed butter and sugar mixture alternately in three parts until the batter is smooth. Spread the batter evenly in the prepared pan. Bake for 30–35 minutes until the cake is golden brown and a cake tester or toothpick comes out clean.

5. **While the cake is baking, make the glaze:** Melt the butter, the remaining 2 tablespoons of orange juice, and the marmalade together in a bowl in the microwave or in a small saucepan set over medium heat.

6. When the cake is done, remove it immediately from the pan onto a serving plate and pour the glaze over the hot cake. Cool and dust with confectioner's sugar right before serving if desired.

Prepare-Ahead Tip: *The cake can be made up to twenty-four hours ahead and kept, loosely covered, at room temperature.*

Cream Scones with Golden Raisins

[photograph 2 1]

This is a teatime classic at the Inn. Whether you indulge in these while sitting on an Adirondack chair looking out over Lake Champlain, curled up in an armchair in front of the library fire at the Inn, or in your own home, be assured that they in no way resemble those dried-out bricks some people dare to call scones.

◇ *Makes: 24 small triangular scones*

3 cups all-purpose flour

½ cup sugar plus additional for sprinkling scone tops

1 tablespoon baking powder

½ teaspoon table salt

¾ cup (1½ sticks) cold unsalted butter, cut into small cubes

2 large eggs

1 cup heavy cream plus additional for brushing scone tops

1 cup golden raisins

Before You Start   You can vary the scones by using other fruits, such as currants; coarsely chopped, sweetened tart cherries; or dried apricots. My favorite is finely diced crystallized ginger.

1. Preheat the oven to 400°F. In a large mixing bowl, whisk together the flour, sugar, baking powder, and salt.

2. With your fingers, two forks, or a pastry blender, work the butter into the flour mixture until most of the dough looks like fine gravel with a few larger butter bumps throughout. (Alternatively, use a food processor with a few short pulses.)

3. In a small bowl, whisk together the eggs and heavy cream. Pour the egg mixture into the flour mixture and stir with a fork to form large, moist clumps of dough. (Or pulse again just a few times.) Stir in the golden raisins.

4. Turn the dough out onto a lightly floured counter and knead it about ten times until it just comes together, taking care not to overwork the dough. The dough will be quite sticky.

5. Divide the dough into three equal portions and pat each into a 5- or 6-inch round about ¾ inch thick. Put the rounds on an ungreased cookie sheet, staggering them to allow a little room to expand. Score each round into eight wedges without cutting all the way through. Brush the scone tops with additional cream and sprinkle them with sugar.

6. Bake for 17–19 minutes until the scones are golden and just barely moist along the score marks. (They will continue to cook a little as they cool.) Cool the scones on a rack and break them apart along the score lines when ready to serve.

> **Tip:** *At the Inn, these scones are sometimes served with a homemade version of clotted cream made by whipping 1 cup of heavy cream with 1 tablespoon of confectioner's sugar until the cream has almost turned to butter.*
>
> **Prepare-Ahead Tip:** *The scone dough can be made ahead, frozen in scored rounds on a cookie sheet, and then popped into zippered plastic bags to store. Take the rounds out of the freezer, preheat the oven, brush the rounds with cream and sprinkle them with sugar, and bake for about 25–28 minutes.*

Staying Small

Carleton Yoder, cheesemaker,
Champlain Valley Creamery

"Why should a fresh cheese last in your fridge for up to a year?"

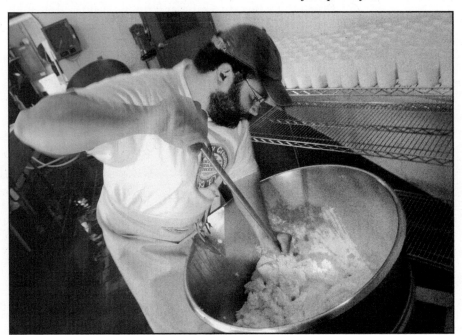

*t*he dirt never quite disappears from the fingernails of a vegetable farmer. By contrast, you can tell cheesemakers by their spotlessly clean hands, which are often red and chafed from perpetual washing.

It is critical to touch the cheese, not only to work with it, but also to feel when it is ready, explains Carleton Yoder as he opens up a bag of curds and gently sinks a finger into the soft, dense mass that is just a step away from cream cheese. "This is the way I like it," he says with satisfaction, and starts lifting out the bags and dumping their contents into a huge stainless steel mixing bowl, pausing once to answer the phone (a restaurant ordering cream cheese for cheesecake) and then wash his hands once again before returning to the bags.

Carleton is Champlain Valley Creamery's owner, milk hauler, cheesemaker, salesman, and often the delivery guy too. He has another part-time sales job, and he still waits tables sometimes. ("I'm obviously not doing this for the money," he grins.) A self-described "fermented food nerd," he worked for a hard cider maker in Vermont and then—when he decided to try his hand at lactic fermentation—he spent a season as a cheesemaker at Shelburne Farms. "You can read all the books you want, but it's not like doing it," he says. "And even though they're big compared to what I'm doing, Shelburne Farms is still small scale."

Yesterday morning he hauled sixty gallons of fresh, organic milk from Journey's Hope Farm in nearby Bridport back to the huge, old, brick building in Vergennes where he has made cheese since late 2003. Although Carleton's neighbors are now mostly tourist knickknack shops, the space has a history he appreciates. It was originally built in 1909 as a creamery along the old railroad line, where local farmers would drop off their milk for bottling and shipping. In his small, second-floor cheeseroom, milk is once again being processed: it is separated, pasteurized, and cooled, and then rennet and culture are added. After the milk and cream mixture gets "as thick as yogurt," he scoops the curds into nylon muslin bags and stacks them on top of each other so that their own weight slowly pushes out excess liquid until they reach perfect cream cheese consistency. After a brief mixing with salt, the cheese is ready to be packed into tubs.

The relatively simple process yields mild, soft, creamy, spreadable cheese that bears only a passing resemblance to the gummy mainstream version. "It's an artisan twist on a very familiar industrial cheese, made the way cream cheese was once," Carleton says. "It's local and organic, with no stabilizers or preservatives. Why should a fresh cheese last in your fridge for up to a year?"

Cream cheese was a good option for a cheese start-up, Carleton explains as he stirs salt with a giant stainless steel paddle into the cream cheese, which is soft and light like a good sponge cake batter. "I thought it was something I could do by myself," he says. Cash flow, while still slow, is steady because the cheese can be sold right away. He's experimenting with some other cheeses too: a small triple-cream that is aged for ten days and ricotta salata made with leftover skim milk. It would be nice if he could quit his other jobs, he says, but he doesn't plan to get too much bigger. "I try to do things traditionally," he says, "and I want to keep it small."

Maple–Cream Cheese Pound Cake

This is a classic cream cheese pound cake with a dense, moist texture to which we added the extra Vermont touch of deep maple flavor. In the summer we top slices with fresh blueberries and grilled peaches brushed with a little maple syrup. A dollop of crème fraîche swirled with a little maple syrup finishes the plate perfectly. In the fall or winter, layer cubes of the cake in the Roasted Apple and Plum Parfaits (page 221). A nice slice of cake is also great just by itself with a cup of tea or coffee.
◇ *Makes: two 8½ by 4½-inch or 9 by 5-inch loaves*

8 ounces cream cheese, very soft

1½ cups (3 sticks) unsalted butter, at room temperature

2 cups granulated white sugar

1 cup granulated maple sugar, sifted or buzzed in a food processor to remove large lumps (see Before You Start)

1 teaspoon table salt

1 tablespoon pure maple syrup

6 large eggs

3 cups all-purpose flour

Before You Start   The cream cheese must be very soft in order to make a smooth batter, so give it plenty of time to soften. Of course, we love to use Champlain Valley Creamery fresh cream cheese, which makes the pound cakes extra rich and dense, but the recipe will work fine with regular cream cheese. Maple sugar and syrup do speed up browning, so watch the pound cakes carefully and tent them with foil if the tops get too dark before they are baked through. For the same reason, you will have the best results with glass or lighter colored pans, as dark pans also hasten browning. But if the cakes get a little crusty on the outside, don't worry; people have been known to fight over those end slices. If you can't find maple sugar in a store near you, see Sources (page 273) or substitute light brown sugar.

1. Preheat the oven to 325°F. Generously butter the loaf pans.

2. In the bowl of a standing mixer fitted with the paddle attachment, beat together the cream cheese and butter until they are completely smooth, 4–5 minutes. Scrape down the sides and bottom of the bowl. Add the white and maple sugars and salt and continue to beat until light and fluffy, 5 more minutes, stopping once or twice to scrape down the bowl.

3. In a medium bowl, whisk together the maple syrup and eggs. With the mixer running on low speed, gradually add the egg mixture to the cream cheese mixture, making sure each addition is incorporated before adding more. Scrape down the bowl. Add the flour 1 cup at a time, mixing on low until it is all incorporated. Scrape down the bowl and beat for 1 more minute until the batter is completely smooth.

4. Divide the batter evenly between the pans and smooth the tops with a spatula. Bake for 35 minutes and then turn the oven down to 300°F and bake for another 45–50 minutes, tenting the tops of the loaves with foil if they get too dark. The cakes are done when a cake tester comes out clean and the crack in the top of the loaf is just barely moist. Remove the cakes immediately from the pans and cool them on a rack.

> **Prepare-Ahead Tip:** *Like most pound cakes, this one holds up beautifully in a sealed container at room temperature for up to a week. It also freezes very well.*

Hot Milk Sponge Cake

[photograph 22]

This is a New England staple, a recipe handed down by grandmothers back when people still baked from scratch. It was an everyday cake if served plain (maybe with a dusting of powdered sugar) but could also be dressed up for special occasions with fresh strawberries and softly whipped cream. ◇ **Makes: one 13 by 9-inch cake or two 9-inch round layers**

2 cups all-purpose flour

2 teaspoons baking powder

1 teaspoon table salt

4 large eggs

2 cups granulated white sugar

1 cup whole or 2 percent milk

2 tablespoons unsalted butter

2 teaspoons pure vanilla extract

Before You Start Make sure you have the oven preheated and waiting for the cake, because the batter deflates if it has to wait.

1. Preheat the oven to 350°F. Butter and flour the pan(s). In a medium bowl, whisk together the flour, baking powder, and salt. Set aside.

2. In the bowl of a standing mixer fitted with the whisk attachment, beat the eggs until light, about 3–4 minutes. With the mixer running on medium, slowly add the sugar and beat until the mixture is light yellow and comes off the whisk in a ribbon when the whisk is lifted, about 7–8 minutes.

3. While the eggs and sugar are beating, bring the milk and butter just to a boil in a small saucepan set over medium heat. (Alternatively, combine them in a small bowl and microwave for about 3 minutes.) Stir the vanilla into the hot milk.

4. With the mixer running on medium speed, slowly add the hot milk mixture to the egg mixture. Mix until combined and then reduce the mixer speed and add the flour mixture slowly, just until thoroughly combined, stopping to scrape down the bowl once or twice. Pour the batter immediately into the prepared pan(s) and place them in oven. (The batter will have bubbles.)

5. Bake the 13 by 9-inch cake for 25–30 minutes or the 9-inch rounds for 20–25 minutes, until the edges are browned and just pulling away from the pan or a cake tester or toothpick comes out clean. Do not overbake.

6. Serve with whipped cream and strawberries as desired.

Variation If you want to make individual strawberry shortcakes, bake the batter in muffin cups for 15–18 minutes.

From the Archives Milk was always in abundant supply at Shelburne Farms. It was even fed to favored household pets, as reported in a letter to the dairyman in 1906: "Please let Breeding Barns have four quarts milk daily for Mrs. Webb's dog." When the Webbs were away from the Farm, milk and cream were shipped to them regularly. In a telegram shortly after they sold their Fifth Avenue home in 1913, Seward Webb apprised his farm manager, "Mrs. Webb and I moved to the Plaza Hotel Wednesday. Will you send three quarts of milk daily to the Plaza Hotel until further orders."

Chocolate–Sour Cream Cake with Bittersweet Chocolate Frosting

[photograph 21]

This is not a cake for children. Although youngsters have been known to gobble it up, it was not designed for their more typically milk chocolate tastes. It was created for people who like their chocolate with a deep, dark, sophisticated edge. The frosting, particularly, delivers a distinctly bittersweet note, along with the tang of sour cream. We love it that way, but if you're looking for a multigenerational crowd pleaser, you may want to use semisweet chocolate in the frosting. Try this topped with Fresh Mint Ice Cream (page 252). ◇ **Makes: one 8- or 9-inch round cake**

For the cake

¼ cup plus 1 teaspoon unsweetened cocoa powder

1 cup all-purpose flour

1½ teaspoons baking powder

¼ teaspoon baking soda

½ teaspoon table salt

2 large eggs

⅓ cup sour cream, not nonfat

1 teaspoon pure vanilla extract

4 ounces coarsely chopped bittersweet chocolate (see Before You Start)

½ cup (1 stick) unsalted butter, cut into 8 pieces

1 cup sugar

⅓ cup hot tap water

Before You Start   Look for a bittersweet chocolate with not more than 60 percent cacao solids for this cake and frosting. The recipe works fine with either natural or Dutch-processed cocoa.

1. Preheat the oven to 325°F with a rack in the lower third of the oven. Prepare an 8-inch round, 2-inch-deep springform cake pan by generously buttering the bottom and sides and placing a circle of parchment in the bottom. Use the teaspoon of cocoa powder to dust the sides of the pan, and shake out any excess.

2. Prepare the cake: In a large bowl, sift together the remaining cocoa powder, flour, baking powder, baking soda, and salt. In a small bowl, whisk together the eggs, sour cream, and vanilla.

3. In a medium bowl in the microwave (see the Tip on page 247) or in the top of a double boiler set over simmering water, melt the chocolate, butter, and sugar with the hot water just until they whisk smoothly together.

4 ounces coarsely chopped bittersweet or semisweet chocolate

1 tablespoon unsalted butter

1 cup sour cream, not nonfat, at room temperature

¾ cup sifted confectioner's sugar

4. Whisk the egg and sour cream mixture into the dry ingredients. Then stir in the chocolate mixture until the batter is smooth. Pour the batter into the prepared pan. Tap the pan once on the counter to remove any air bubbles and bake for about 40–45 minutes until the edges are just pulling away from the sides of the pan and a cake tester or toothpick comes out clean. (The top of the cake may still look a little moist, and if it has cracked, don't worry, because the frosting will happily cover that up.) Run a knife around the side of the pan and release the springform collar. Set the cake on a rack to cool.

5. *When the cake is completely cool, prepare the frosting:* In a medium bowl in the microwave (see the Tip below) or in the top of a double boiler set over simmering water, melt the chocolate and butter just until they whisk together smoothly. Cool the chocolate mixture for 5 minutes and then whisk in the sour cream and confectioner's sugar until smooth. Immediately frost the top and sides of the cake.

Tip: *A microwave can be a great tool for melting chocolate, but its power is so variable that it is hard to give specific directions and you risk burning the chocolate. Always err on the conservative side; very often a mixture will not look melted, but if you whisk it vigorously the residual heat will melt remaining lumps. As a rule of thumb, start with 30 seconds at full power for the first ounce of chocolate and add 10 seconds for each additional ounce of chocolate, taking it out to stir after the first 30 seconds to check how it's doing.*

Prepare-Ahead Tip: *The cake can be baked and frosted a day ahead and kept in a cool, dry place.*

Sweet Milk

Cup Custards with Pears Poached in Sweet Wine

This delicate, old-fashioned dessert was inspired by the 1924 handwritten recipe book of Frederica Webb Pulitzer, Lila and Seward Webb's eldest daughter. Within its pages, I found a recipe for preserved pears closely followed by one for a baked custard, and I thought the two would go well together—especially if the pears were bathed in some lovely dessert wine made from grapes grown right on Shelburne Farms, with a view that Frederica herself might have enjoyed. A few fresh raspberries sprinkled on top of each cup add a nice touch of color or, for a little crunch, add some shards of Maple-Almond Brittle (page 270). ◇ **Serves: 6**

For the pears

¾ cup sweet dessert wine (see Before You Start)

1 tablespoon honey

2 medium, ripe but firm, preferably red-skinned pears such as Red Anjou, quartered lengthwise, then each quarter cored and cut into 4 thin wedges

For the custard

3 large eggs

2 cups whole milk

½ cup granulated white sugar

1 teaspoon pure vanilla extract

¼ teaspoon table salt

Before You Start Mixing the custard in a blender (a modern addition to Frederica's recipe) means you don't have to strain it, but fill the custard cups immediately after blending or the sugar tends to sink to the bottom. Vermont has a number of wineries, including Shelburne Vineyard, an independent business with vineyards on Shelburne Farms. Among its wines are some delicious, sweet, late harvest and ice wines, like the Rhapsody late harvest blend, made with grapes that have truly experienced a Vermont chill (see Sources, page 273). Red-skinned pears add nice color to the dessert; green pears will work fine, although you may want to peel them.

1. Preheat the oven to 325°F. Set six small (6-ounce) ramekins or custard cups in a large baking dish.

2. In a small baking dish, whisk together the dessert wine and honey. Add the pears and toss gently to coat. Cover with foil and set aside.

3. Combine the eggs, milk, sugar, vanilla, and salt in a blender or food processor and blend them together until smooth. Pour the mixture immediately into the custard cups. Pour hot tap water into the baking dish around the cups up to the level of the custard.

4. Carefully place the baking dish of custards into the oven with the baking dish of pears next to it. Bake for 40–45 minutes until the custard is just set and the pears are just tender. (The custard will still jiggle, but when you tip one to the side, it will not run.) Remove the custards carefully from the hot water and set them on a rack to cool. Serve the custards at room temperature topped with the poached pears and their juices.

Sour Cherry–Chocolate Cheesecakes

[photograph 21]

These individual, no-bake cheesecakes combine rich Vermont dairy with the tart sour cherries that come into season for an all-too-brief two weeks each July. Oh yes, there's a little chocolate in there too. ◇ **Makes: 12 cupcake-size individual cheesecakes or 24 mini bite-size cheesecakes**

For the crust

⅔ cup (about 3 ounces) whole raw almonds

2 tablespoons granulated white sugar

2 tablespoons unsalted butter

3 ounces bittersweet chocolate, coarsely chopped

For the sour cherry topping

About 1 pound fresh or frozen pitted sour cherries (2–3 cups) or 1 (14½-ounce) can pitted red tart cherries, drained with juice reserved

1–1½ cups granulated white sugar to taste

Slurry made from either ¼ cup water (for fresh or frozen cherries) or ½ cup juice from can (for canned cherries) whisked with 2 tablespoons cornstarch

For the cheesecake filling

¼ cup heavy cream

2 tablespoons confectioner's sugar

6 ounces cream cheese, very soft

Before You Start   Since the season for fresh sour cherries is fleeting, you are more likely to find frozen sour cherries. If those are not available, canned Montmorency cherries can be found in many supermarkets. The cheesecakes need at least 1 hour to set in the freezer, and can be stored in the freezer for several weeks. When you're ready to serve, thaw them for an hour in the refrigerator or for 30 minutes at cool room temperature. The mini size will thaw more quickly. Since they are not baked, they soften up if left sitting out, which doesn't hurt the flavor but can make eating the larger size a little messy.

1. Set cupcake liners in cupcake or muffin pans or use the stand-alone foil kind set on a cookie sheet. (If you're making bite-size cheesecakes, you'll need half-ounce paper candy cups set in mini-muffin pans.)

2. Prepare the crust: Toast the almonds until fragrant—about 7 minutes at 350°F in a toaster oven or oven. Cool for 5 minutes. In the bowl of a food processor, grind the almonds with the sugar for about 30 seconds until finely ground but not turning into paste.

3. In a medium bowl in the microwave or set on top of a pot of simmering water, melt together the butter and chopped chocolate until smooth. (See the Tip on page 247.) Mix the ground almond mixture into the melted chocolate mixture and, working quickly before it sets, press about 2 teaspoons of the crust into the bottom of each cupcake liner (or 1 teaspoon into each candy cup). Place the crusts in the freezer.

4. *Prepare the cherry topping:* In a medium saucepan set over medium heat, combine the sour cherries with the sugar and the cornstarch slurry. Bring the mixture just to a boil, cook for 30–60 seconds until the liquid thickens, taste for sweetness and add more sugar as desired, then set aside to cool. If using canned cherries, bring the sugar and cornstarch slurry to a boil per above, take the pan off the heat, stir in the cherries, and taste for sweetness. Set aside to cool.

5. *Prepare the filling:* In the bowl of a standing mixer fitted with the whisk attachment, beat the heavy cream with the confectioner's sugar until it holds soft peaks. Scoop it out into another medium bowl.

6. In the same mixer bowl fitted with the paddle attachment, beat together the cream cheese and 2 tablespoons of the liquid from the cooled cherry topping (without any cherries) until smooth. Using a spatula, fold the whipped cream into the cream cheese mixture.

7. Remove the chilled crusts from the freezer. Fill each crust with 1 tablespoon of the cheesecake filling (1 generous teaspoon for the candy cup size) and smooth the top. Dollop 3–4 cherries on top (2–3 for candy cup size) with a little liquid. (If you have any left over, it's great over ice cream or in yogurt.)

8. Cover the cheesecakes with foil or plastic wrap and return them to the freezer for at least one hour and up to several weeks. See Before You Start on page 250 for serving instructions.

Fresh Mint Ice Cream

This recipe has become a favorite during Shelburne Farms camps, when the young participants actually gather many of the ingredients themselves from all over the Farm: mint from the gardens, milk and cream from the dairy, eggs from the chickens in the Children's Farmyard, and honey from hives on the property (well, they don't actually collect that, but they see it at the source). The resulting ice cream doesn't have the same otherworldly, bright green tint as the mint ice cream they might be used to, but that doesn't seem to prevent them from slurping it all up.

◇ *Makes: about 1 quart*

⅔ cup loosely packed fresh mint leaves

¾ cup granulated white sugar

2½ cups whole milk

1½ cups heavy cream

4 large egg yolks

¼ cup honey

¼ teaspoon table salt

¾ teaspoon pure vanilla extract

Before You Start Many hands make light work grinding the mint and sugar together during camp, but unless you have lots of eager helpers, you may find a food processor handy for that task. And, no, cacao doesn't grow on the Farm, but a cupful of mini chocolate chips stirred in at the end might be a nice addition. The campers sometimes top their scoops with fresh strawberries from the gardens or even wild raspberries they've picked earlier in the day.

1. Place the mint leaves and sugar in a bowl and grind the leaves into the sugar with a pestle or cup. (Alternatively, process the mint and sugar together in a food processor until the mint is finely ground.)

2. In a medium saucepan, heat the milk and cream over medium heat, stirring occasionally. Whisk the egg yolks in a medium bowl until smooth, then add the sugar and mint mixture and whisk until combined. When the milk mixture steams and is hot but not simmering, whisk ¼ cup of the hot milk mixture into the egg mixture. Then whisk in another ¼ cup of the hot milk mixture. Take the saucepan off the heat and stir the now tempered egg mixture into the milk mixture.

3. Put the saucepan back over medium heat and add the honey and salt. Cook, stirring, until the mixture is thick enough that a line drawn by your finger across a coated spoon leaves a mark, about 5 minutes. Do not allow the mixture to boil. Stir in the vanilla.

4. Cool the custard quickly by setting the saucepan in an ice bath and stirring it for a few minutes. Cover and refrigerate until thoroughly chilled, at least 1 hour and up to 24 hours.

5. When you're ready to make the ice cream, pour the chilled custard through a fine sieve to remove the mint leaves and freeze in your ice cream maker according to the manufacturer's instructions.

Buttermilk-Plum Sherbet

[*photograph 23*]

This was inspired by a bushel of small, deep pink–red Waneta plums from a Market-Garden tree, whose amazing, sweet, apricot-tinted flesh and luminous, rosy pink skin made a gorgeous blushing sherbet. Part of the charm of this recipe is seeing and tasting how the results differ with each type of plum, and it's fun to serve different batches together to showcase the diversity. We've used everything from heirloom Kirk's Blue plums to tiny Damsons to the widely available Italian prune plum. Whatever variety you use, the sherbet goes beautifully with Maple Gingersnaps (page 262). For an elegant but fun dessert, have guests make their own ice cream sandwiches. ◇ ***Makes: 1 quart***

1½ pounds ripe plums, halved and pitted

½ cup granulated white sugar

½ cup honey plus more to taste

1½ cups buttermilk

Freshly squeezed lemon juice to taste (optional)

Before You Start Any variety of plum will work in this recipe—just make sure they are very ripe. In fact, this is the perfect opportunity to use fruit that may be just a bit overripe. The relative sweetness or tartness of the end result will, of course, depend on the fruit, but you can adjust the honey or add lemon juice to taste. This recipe works best with an ice cream maker, although it can also be made by freezing the mixture in a deep pot, then using a handheld electric mixer to churn it every hour for about three hours.

1. Put the plums, sugar, and honey in a medium saucepan over medium heat and bring to a simmer. Simmer for 10–20 minutes until the fruit is completely broken down. (The time can vary widely depending on the variety and ripeness of the plums.)

2. Run the plum mixture through a food mill—or press it through a colander to catch the skins—into a large bowl. Stir in the buttermilk. Taste and add a little more honey if the mixture is too tart or a little fresh lemon juice if it's too sweet. Cool and then refrigerate for at least 3 hours, preferably overnight.

3. Freeze in your ice cream maker according to the manufacturer's instructions, or try the alternate freezing procedure detailed in Before You Start.

Sweet Maple

- Maple-Nut Granola
- Streuseled Maple Corn Muffins
- Maple-Butterscotch Pudding
- Maple Gingersnaps
- Maple Sugar Blondies
- Maple-Walnut Pie Squares
- Maple-Almond Brittle
- Maple-Butterscotch Sauce

*[See A Note on Maple, **page 38**, for more information on cooking with maple.]*

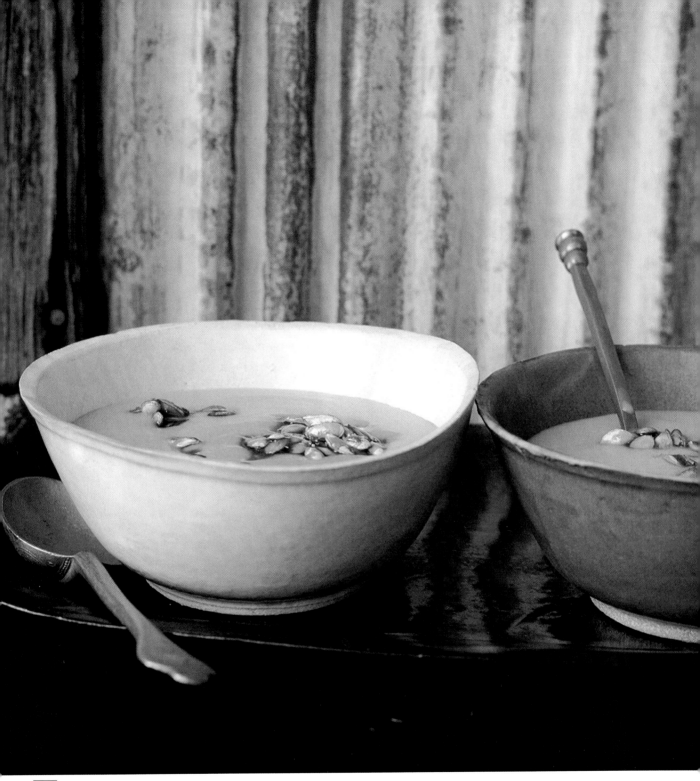

Maple-Roasted Butternut Squash Puree or Soup *(page 202)* with Maple-Glazed Squash Seeds *(page 42)*

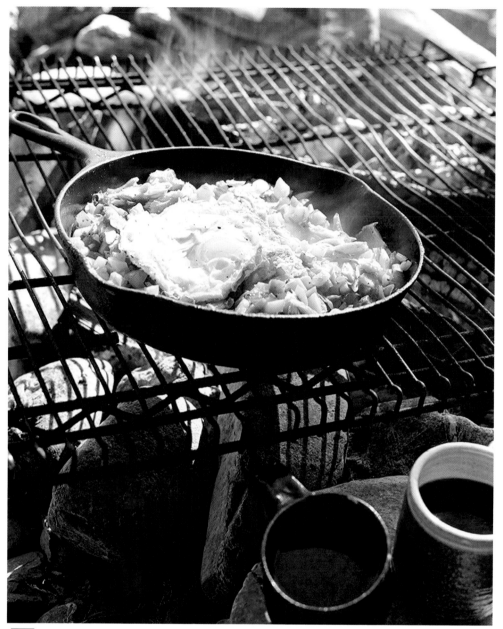

Golden Flannel
Hash *(page 204)*

Opposite: Roasted Apple and
Plum Parfaits *(page 221)* with
Maple-Almond Brittle *(page 270)*

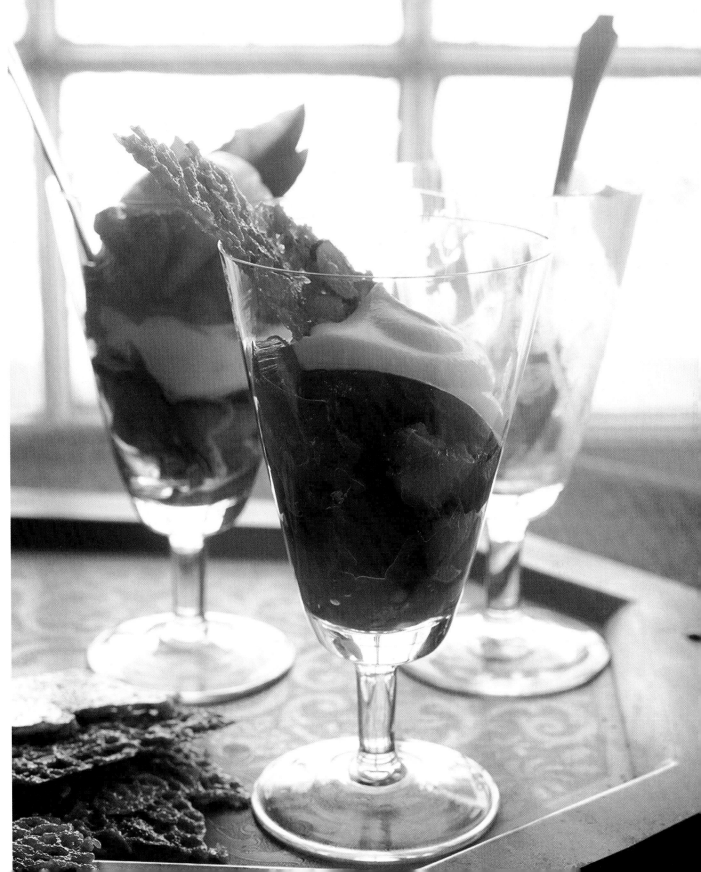

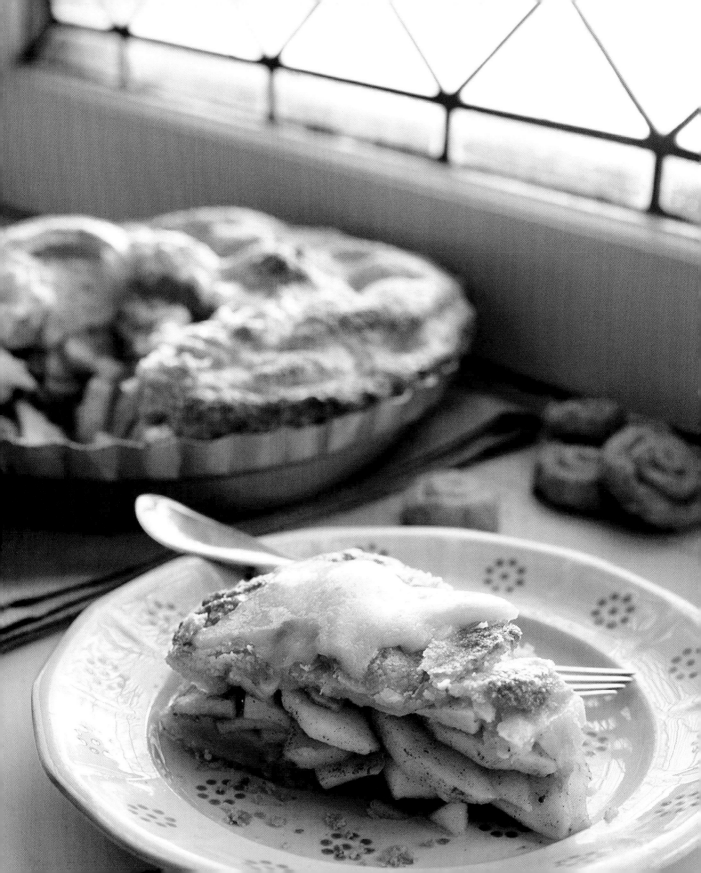

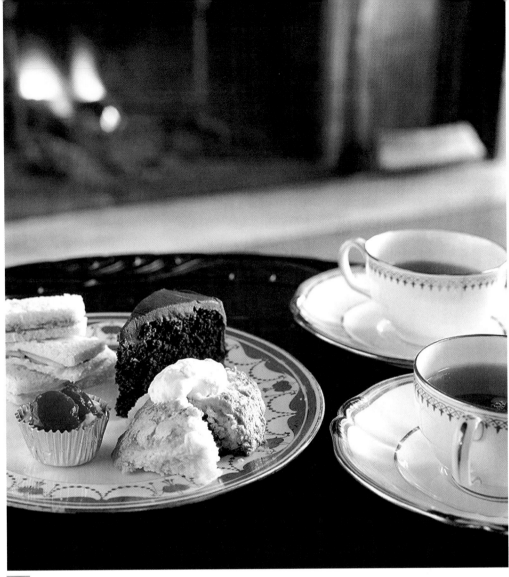

21

Tea plate: Chocolate–Sour Cream Cake with Bittersweet Chocolate Frosting *(page 246)*, Cream Scones with Golden Raisins *(page 238)*, Sour Cherry–Chocolate Cheesecakes *(page 250)*, and Deviled Ham and Cheddar Spread *(page 168)*

Opposite: Apple Pie and Cinnamon Pinwheels *(page 226)*

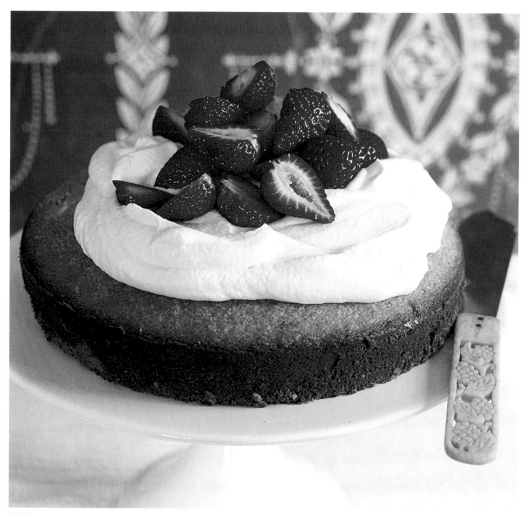

Hot Milk Sponge Cake *(page 244)*

Opposite: Buttermilk–Plum Sherbet *(page 254)*
with Maple Gingersnaps *(page 262)*

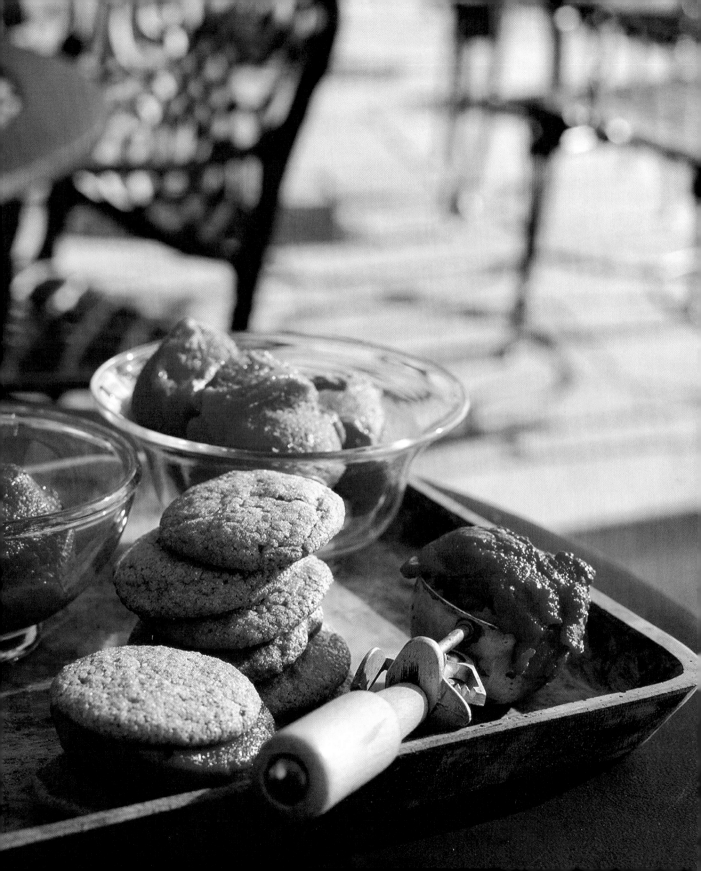

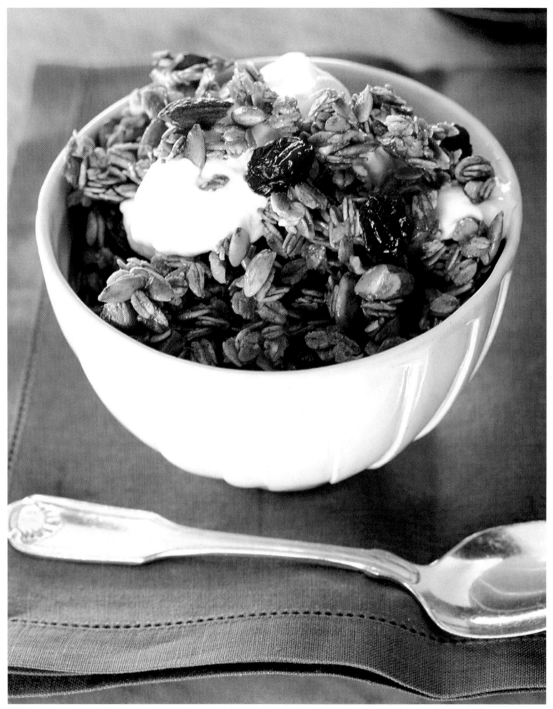

Maple-Nut Granola *(page 258)*

*t*he smell of a sugarhouse is good enough to eat by itself, but the hours it takes to boil down every forty gallons of barely sugary sap into one gallon of liquid gold give sugarmakers plenty of time to dream up ways to enjoy the results of their labor. On the sweet end of the spectrum, local maple festivals feature everything from maple cotton candy to maple fudge to layer cakes festooned with swirls of boiled maple frosting.

Most sugarmakers, though, are purists, preferring fresh syrup stirred into their coffee, drizzled over ice cream, puddling around a stack of pancakes, or captured in the crevices of a waffle. Wherever maple is used, it adds something beyond sweetness. It brings just a hint of the earth from which it comes.

Of course, the quintessential way to enjoy the season's new batch of syrup is at sugar-on-snow parties held across the state in late March and early April, usually near a steaming, smoky sugarhouse. For sugar on snow, syrup is boiled to the point where it solidifies into a soft, chewy, taffylike consistency when it hits a scoop of fresh snow. The traditional accompaniment is a nice big sour pickle, a tradition of mysterious origin best explained perhaps, as an old Vermont cookbook put it: "The pickles are served so that you can eat more sugar."

Maple-Nut Granola

[photograph 24]

Granola is easy to make and fun to customize with your choice of seeds, nuts, and dried fruit. Store-bought ones always seem stingy on the nuts and fruit to me, so I load mine up. ◇ **Makes: about 7 cups (can easily be doubled; see Tip, page 259)**

¼ cup vegetable oil

¼ cup pure maple syrup, Grade B for strongest flavor

¼ cup honey

1 tablespoon granulated maple sugar or light brown sugar

1 teaspoon ground cinnamon

¼ teaspoon table salt

3 cups old-fashioned oats (quick-cooking are fine, but not instant)

1 cup raw, hulled pumpkin seeds (also known as pepitas) or raw sunflower seeds

1 cup natural slivered, sliced, or roughly chopped whole natural almonds or other nut of your choice, such as cashews, pecans, or pistachios

2 cups sweetened dried cherries or cranberries

Before You Start   We like our granola to have clumps and find we get the most by using some honey, turning the mixture carefully just once during cooking rather than stirring, and letting it cool completely before touching it. Just a pinch of salt really brings out the other flavors.

1. Preheat the oven to 350°F. Line a 15 by 10-inch rimmed cookie sheet or shallow roasting pan with a nonstick baking mat or parchment paper. In a small bowl, stir together the oil, syrup, honey, maple sugar, cinnamon, and salt.

2. In a large bowl, mix together the oats, pumpkin seeds, and almonds. Pour the wet mixture over the oat mixture and toss until evenly coated. Spread the granola evenly in the prepared pan. Bake for 15–20 minutes until deep golden brown.

3. Reduce the oven temperature to 300°F and leave the oven door ajar to bring the temperature down while you use a spatula to gently turn the granola, trying not to break up clumps. Bake for another 8–10 minutes until the granola is toasty brown, but watch carefully to make sure it doesn't burn.

4. Set the pan on a wire cooling rack and do not touch the granola until it has completely cooled. Break it into desired size clumps and mix in the dried cherries. Store in an airtight container.

Variation Try changing your dried fruit seasonally like Shelburne Farms employee Tammy Long and her husband Geof do with the Green Mountain Granola they make for the Inn and other customers. They mix in dried blueberries during the summer, apples in the fall, and cranberries with apricots for the holidays.

> **Tip:** *You can double the recipe and make two pans at once. Switch the pans between the upper and lower racks halfway through the higher-temperature baking time, and add a few minutes to both baking phases.*

Sweet Maple

Streuseled Maple Corn Muffins

With their sweet, crunchy topping, these muffins are great for breakfast, brunch, or a midmorning snack. They also work well without the streusel as a lightly sweet corn muffin to eat with our Venison Chili (page 152), or use them for the Pork Loin with Pear and Cornbread Stuffing (page 179). ◇ *Makes: 12 muffins*

For the streusel topping

2 tablespoons all-purpose flour

2 tablespoons pure maple syrup

1 tablespoon unsalted butter, at room temperature

¼ cup finely chopped pecans

For the muffins

1½ cups all-purpose flour

½ cup fine cornmeal, white or yellow

1½ teaspoons baking powder

½ teaspoon baking soda

½ teaspoon table salt

¼ cup (½ stick) unsalted butter

½ cup pure maple syrup, Grade B for strongest flavor

½ cup sour cream, not nonfat

½ cup milk

2 large eggs

Before You Start   Although we normally prefer using locally grown, stone-ground cornmeal, it makes these muffins a little too heavy, so we've gone with the fine cornmeal found easily on most supermarket shelves.

1. Preheat the oven to 375°F. Generously grease a twelve-cup muffin pan or use paper liners.

2. *Make the streusel topping*: In a small bowl, combine the flour, maple syrup, butter, and pecans and mix together with a fork or your fingers. Set aside.

3. *Make the muffins*: In a large bowl, whisk together the flour, cornmeal, baking powder, baking soda, and salt. In a medium bowl in the microwave or in a medium pot set over medium heat, melt the butter. Off the heat, stir in the maple syrup, sour cream, milk, and eggs, in that order, until fully blended.

4. Gradually add the wet mixture to the dry mixture, stirring just until combined but not completely smooth. Do not overmix or your muffins will be tough.

5. Fill the muffin cups about ¾ full with batter and top with a generous teaspoon of streusel, pressing it in gently if necessary.

6. Bake the muffins for about 17–20 minutes until they are golden and a cake tester or toothpick comes out clean. Remove immediately from the pan to cool on a rack.

Maple-Butterscotch Pudding

Forget all about that boxed tan stuff that passes for butterscotch pudding these days. This is the real thing with a light maple-butterscotch flavor and a deep creaminess that you'll want to dive right into. For an adult twist, try the sophisticated coffee variation sprinkled with some chopped, toasted hazelnuts. There are also those who would argue for a dollop of unsweetened whipped cream on top. ◇ ***Serves: 6***

¼ cup (½ stick) unsalted butter

½ cup packed light brown sugar

½ cup pure maple syrup, Grade B for strongest flavor

⅛ teaspoon table salt

2¼ cups half-and-half

3 large egg yolks, lightly beaten

3 tablespoons cornstarch

Before You Start   This recipe moves quickly, so it is important to have your ingredients measured out and equipment ready before beginning.

1. In a medium, heavy-bottomed saucepan, melt the butter over medium heat. Take the pan briefly off the heat and whisk in the brown sugar. Put the pan back on the heat and whisk in the maple syrup and salt. Cook 1–2 minutes, just until foamy.

2. Take the pan off the heat and whisk in the half-and-half. (Be careful because it may spatter.) Put the pan back over medium heat and bring to a simmer. Pull the pan off the heat.

3. Gradually whisk about ½ cup of the hot half-and-half mixture into the beaten egg yolks to temper them. Whisk the cornstarch into the warm egg yolk mixture until dissolved.

4. Put the pan back over medium-low heat and, whisking constantly, gradually pour the egg yolk mixture into the pan.

5. Cook, continuing to whisk constantly, just until the mixture thickens, about 1–2 minutes, or until the first bubble appears.

6. Pour the pudding through a sieve into a serving bowl or six small (6-ounce) ramekins or custard cups. Chill uncovered until set, at least 2 hours.

Variation For a nice counterpoint to the maple sweetness, stir in 1–2 tablespoons of cold, strong coffee, to taste, right before passing the pudding through the sieve.

Maple Gingersnaps

[photograph 23]

This recipe is adapted from one created by a former chef at the Inn, Tom Bivins, who was inspired by some wild ginger found by wildcrafters Nova Kim and Les Hook (see "Wild Mushrooms" chapter). There has been some controversy about whether we can call these gingersnaps, because they are chewy and don't snap, but they're delicious, whatever you call them. ◇ **Makes: about thirty-six 2-inch cookies**

2¼ cups all-purpose flour

2 teaspoons ground ginger (see Before You Start)

½ teaspoon ground allspice

1 teaspoon ground cinnamon

2 teaspoons baking soda

½ teaspoon salt

¼ teaspoon ground white pepper

¾ cup granulated white sugar

½ cup light brown sugar

1 cup (2 sticks) unsalted butter, at room temperature

1 large egg

¼ cup plus 2 tablespoons pure maple syrup, Grade B for strongest flavor

Before You Start   If you can forage some ground wild ginger from an herbal store (see Sources, page 273), it adds an amazing floral note to the cookies, but they are also wonderful with regular ginger, which is actually from a different family of plants altogether. Don't skip the white pepper; it adds a distinctive and delightful little kick. You can refrigerate the dough for longer than 30 minutes and then let it sit at room temperature until you can work easily with it. If it's too cold, the cookies won't spread like they're supposed to.

1. In a medium bowl, whisk together the flour, ginger, allspice, cinnamon, baking soda, salt, and white pepper.

2. In the bowl of a standing mixer fitted with the paddle attachment, combine ½ cup of the white sugar, the brown sugar, and the butter. Cream on medium speed for two minutes or until the mixture is light and fluffy. Stop to scrape down the sides of the bowl at least once. With the mixer running on medium, add the egg and then the maple syrup.

3. With the mixer on slow speed, add the dry ingredients and mix thoroughly. Refrigerate the dough for at least 30 minutes and preheat the oven to 325°F.

4. Roll the dough into ¾-inch balls and roll them in the remaining ¼ cup white sugar. Bake the cookies on a lightly greased or parchment-lined cookie sheet, 3–4 inches apart, for about 15 minutes, until golden brown and set at the edges but still soft in the middle. Cool the cookies for 5 minutes before removing them to a cooling rack.

Variation One of our testers had the inspired idea to stir some finely chopped crystallized ginger into the batter to really heighten the ginger flavor.

Maple Sugar Blondies

The Inn's pastry team created these supersweet, buttery bars for a special maple-themed dinner, and they knocked everyone's socks off. ◇ **Makes: 24 bars**

For the blondie base

2¼ cups all-purpose flour

1 teaspoon baking soda

½ teaspoon table salt

¾ cup canola oil

¼ cup pure maple syrup, Grade B for strongest flavor

¾ cups granulated maple sugar (see Before You Start)

¼ cup granulated white sugar

1 large egg, beaten

For the frosting

¼ cup pure maple syrup, Grade B for strongest flavor

½ cup granulated maple sugar (see Before You Start)

½ cup confectioner's sugar

6 tablespoons cold unsalted butter, cut into small pieces

½ teaspoon pure vanilla extract

Before You Start Maple sugar can vary in texture from quite fine to fairly lumpy. Sift it or buzz it in a food processor to get it as fine as possible. If you can't find maple sugar, substitute packed light brown sugar.

1. Preheat the oven to 350°F and lightly grease a 9 by 13-inch baking pan. In a medium bowl, whisk together the flour, baking soda, and salt.

2. Prepare the blondies: In the bowl of a standing mixer fitted with the paddle attachment and set on medium speed, beat together the canola oil, maple syrup, maple sugar, and white sugar until well blended. With the mixer running, add the egg in a slow stream. Finally, mix in the flour mixture on low speed in thirds, blending carefully after each addition.

3. Turn the dough into the prepared pan and press it down evenly. Bake for 20–25 minutes until the blondies are golden brown and starting to crack on the top like brownies. If you touch the middle, it should not jiggle, but it should still be soft like brownies. Remove the pan to a cooling rack and cool for about 30 minutes before frosting. It should be warm to the touch, but not hot.

4. While the blondies are baking, make the frosting: In a medium, heavy-bottomed saucepan, bring the maple syrup to a simmer over medium-high heat. Immediately reduce the heat and simmer gently for 2 minutes. Remove the pan from the heat and whisk in the maple sugar.

5. Pour the warm maple syrup into the bowl of a food processor and add the confectioner's sugar. Process for 30 seconds. Scrape down the sides of the food processor with a spatula, and process for 1 minute more, scraping down the sides again if necessary.

6. Keep the food processor running while adding the butter pieces through the feed tube. Add the vanilla through the tube and process the frosting until it is completely smooth. (If it sets a little while waiting for the blondies, just whir it a few times in the food processor.)

7. Use a spatula to spread the frosting evenly over the warm blondies and cool them completely before cutting.

Variation Some people like to sprinkle finely chopped pecans over the frosting.

Passing It On

"It's all about developing a sense of place and having a greater understanding of our agricultural and natural world."

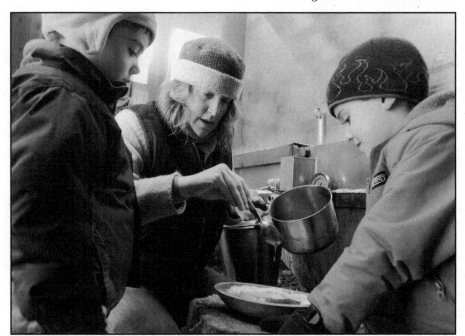

a group of adults is barking at the edge of the Shelburne Farms sugarbush one chilly January day. "We protect the tree. Ruff, (rough), ruff," they chant as they circle others who are role-playing the inner parts of the tree in a slightly quieter way. The scene will repeat itself frequently with younger participants from mid-March through April, when hundreds of students come to the Farm on sugaring field trips to learn about trees, tap maples, collect sap, and breathe in the damp sweetness of a sugarhouse.

Today's workshop attendees include teachers, environmental educators from conservancies and science centers, and sugarmakers, who will take these hands-on educational activities back to three states. Although their students or young visitors may think it's all about syrup, they know that sugaring offers an opportunity to share lessons about woodland ecology and sustainable forestry.

The next activity involves pairs: one partner leads the other to a tree for a sightless encounter. One can imagine giggling grade-schoolers pulling their blindfolded friends astray in the woods, but the workshop leaders offer the educators practical tips for keeping things on track. At their trees, participants reach out and feel the bark, then stretch their arms around the trunk, hands exploring for branches, distinctive knobs, or previous years' maple tap holes. Soft snowflakes start to fall as they are then led back to the starting point and challenged to find that same tree again with their eyes open.

Shelburne Farms offers seasonally themed field trips, camps, and workshops for youngsters, families, and adults throughout the year: animal tracking in the winter, exploring the changing forest in fall, a summer day in the life of a farmer. "It's all about developing a sense of place and having a greater understanding of our agricultural and natural world," says Dana Hudson, an agriculture educator for Shelburne Farms. It's about working with educators to help them meet their goals and also nurture in their students strong and tangible connections with the earth, she continues. "We know that the more actual experiences kids have with something, the more likely they are to value it."

Often the simplest activities have the most impact: realizing that you can find your way back to a tree without ever having seen it, or just lying on your stomach in a field and writing down everything within a circle around you. A tree or a patch of roadside grass that you pass by daily looks different forever if you stop one day and pay a little attention to it. One of the activities is collective poetry writing, in which a small group of students contribute a few words each about a place and then string them together into a poem. "The trees calm me down, the leaves move like they're dancing, everything falls," reads one poem written by fourth- and fifth-graders from an urban elementary school. "A long path for me, flowers fall on me lightly, when I come by slow," goes another.

The ultimate goal is to pass on the message that the earth should be treasured and cared for, but that rarely needs to be said. Just give them the opportunity, says Dana, and "kids will discover that for themselves."

Maple-Walnut Pie Squares

Maple syrup pies are a Vermont tradition, but since pie is more of a special occasion dish for most people, we decided to pour the same maple-sweet, buttery filling over an easy, press-in crust. The best thing is that the bars are finger food, which can't be said about most maple pies. The filling recipe is adapted from one recommended by Dave Marvin and his wife, Lucy, of Butternut Mountain Farm (see "Savory Maple" chapter) and comes from an old friend of theirs, Pauline Couture of Couture's Maple Shop in Westfield. ◇ ***Makes: 12 bars***

For the crust

1¼ cups all-purpose flour

¼ teaspoon baking soda

⅛ teaspoon table salt

½ cup (1 stick) unsalted butter, at room temperature

⅓ cup packed light brown sugar

½ cup finely chopped walnuts

For the filling

2 tablespoons unsalted butter

½ cup pure maple syrup, Grade B for strongest flavor

3 tablespoons packed light brown sugar

⅛ teaspoon table salt

1 large egg

1 cup coarsely chopped walnuts (optional)

Before You Start   Pauline stirs walnuts into her filling; we put the walnuts in the crust instead, but feel free to stir more into your filling.

1. Preheat the oven to 375°F. Generously grease the bottom and sides of a 9 by 9-inch baking pan.

2. *Make the crust*: In a small bowl, whisk together the flour, baking soda, and salt. In the bowl of a standing mixer fitted with the paddle attachment or with a handheld electric mixer, cream together the butter and brown sugar until fluffy. Gradually add the flour mixture in thirds, beating to blend between additions. Finally, mix in the walnuts just until distributed. Pat the crust firmly and evenly into the prepared pan and bake for 8–10 minutes, just until golden.

3. *While the crust is baking, make the topping*: In a medium bowl in the microwave or in a medium pot set over medium heat, melt the butter. Off the heat, whisk in the maple syrup, brown sugar, salt, and egg. Stir in the walnuts, if using.

4. Pour the topping over the hot crust. Return the pan to the oven for 13–15 minutes, until the topping is deep brown and set. Cool completely on a rack before cutting.

From the Archives Back in the original days of Shelburne Farms, Vermont was butternut country, and that's what would have been used in a recipe like this. Old-timers still remember long hours spent cracking the rather stubborn shells, and community cookbooks are filled with recipes for cookies, pies, and sweet breads made with butternuts, also known as white walnuts. Over the last thirty years, a fungus has decimated most of the butternuts across the state—and the country—but a few still stand at Shelburne Farms, and place names like Butternut Hill testify to the presence they once had.

Maple-Almond Brittle

[*photograph* 19]

A crunchy, sweet, and nutty treat to be eaten as candy or crumbled over Roasted Apple and Plum Parfaits (page 221) or Cup Custards with Pears Poached in Sweet Wine (page 248). ◇ **Makes: 3 cups crumbled brittle**

⅓ cup all-purpose flour

¼ teaspoon baking powder

⅛ teaspoon baking soda

⅛ teaspoon table salt

¼ cup (½ stick) unsalted butter

½ cup pure maple syrup, not Grade B

½ cup sliced almonds

Before You Start   The timing on baking this is a little tricky, but it's worth it. You may have to sacrifice a few burned edges to get the middle crunchy.

1. Preheat the oven to 350°F and line a cookie sheet with a nonstick baking mat or parchment paper. In a small bowl, whisk together the flour, baking powder, baking soda, and salt.

2. In a medium saucepan, melt the butter with the maple syrup over medium heat until the mixture comes to a boil. Boil for 1 minute. Take the pan off the heat and immediately whisk in the flour mixture, then stir in the almonds.

3. Using a spatula, spread the batter evenly and thinly onto the prepared cookie sheet in a rough, 12 by 9-inch rectangle. (The outer edge will cook more quickly, so it is especially important to make sure the middle is thin; also make sure you distribute the almonds evenly.)

4. Bake the brittle for about 11–13 minutes until dark golden brown. (The edges may look close to burned, but it needs to go this far or it won't be brittle when cooled.)

5. Cool on a rack and then break into irregular 1- to 2-inch pieces. The brittle will keep for two or three days in a sealed container.

Maple-Butterscotch Sauce

Nothing could be better than pure maple syrup poured over vanilla ice cream—except maybe this sauce. It is also great with ice cream and over our Roasted Apple and Plum Parfaits (page 221). Try it as a dip for crisp apple slices or for a fun fondue dessert with fruit and our Maple–Cream Cheese Pound Cake (page 242). You can also drizzle it hot over fresh snow (or see the purist version below). ◇ **Makes: About 1½ cups sauce**

½ cup granulated maple sugar or packed light brown sugar

½ cup pure maple syrup, not Grade B

½ cup (1 stick) unsalted butter

½ cup heavy cream

Pinch coarse kosher salt

Before You Start   This sauce keeps refrigerated pretty much forever, but you are very unlikely to have it around that long. It will solidify when cool, so either warm it by running the jar under hot water or heat it briefly at 50 percent power in the microwave.

1. In a medium saucepan set over medium heat, melt together the maple sugar, maple syrup, and butter until the sugar is dissolved, whisking frequently.

2. Increase the heat to medium-high and bring the mixture to a boil. Cook, without stirring, for about 4 minutes.

3. Remove the pot from the heat and stir in the cream. (Be careful because it may spatter.) Add the salt and whisk until smooth.

Variation   To make straight-ahead sugar on snow, all you need to do is boil maple syrup in a heavy-bottomed pot over medium-high heat until it reaches 235–238°F, or what is known as "soft-ball" stage. (If you don't have a candy thermometer, another way to see if the syrup has reached the right stage is to pour some on snow, where it should firm up.) Scoop up some fresh snow and drizzle the hot syrup over it. It will turn into chewy maple taffy. To be truly authentic, eat it with a big pickle.

Sources

For Shelburne Farms' award-winning farmhouse cheddar cheese, private-label ham and bacon, maple syrup, honey, fruit preserves, mustards, and other Vermont products:

- Shelburne Farms mail-order catalog: (802) 985-8686
- Shelburne Farms Welcome Center and Farm Store: (802) 985-8442
- Shelburne Farms Web site: www.shelburnefarms.org

Independent producers located on Shelburne Farms:

- O-Bread Bakery: (802) 985-8771 or obread@aol.com
- Shelburne Vineyard: (802) 734-8700 or www.shelburnevineyard.com

For Vermont cheesemakers and their cheeses:

- Vermont Cheese Council: www.vtcheese.com
- Champlain Valley Creamery, Vergennes: (802) 877-2950 or www.cvcream.com

For pure Vermont maple syrup, granulated maple sugar, and other maple products:

- Vermont Maple Sugar Makers' Association and Maple Foundation: www.vermontmaple.org
- Butternut Mountain Farms, Johnson and Morrisville: (802) 888-3491 or (800) 828-2376

For fresh or dried wild mushrooms from Vermont:

- Les Hook and Nova Kim, VT Native, Albany: (802) 755-6286 or www.wildorganicfood.com

For Vermont pork:

- Duclos and Thompson Farm, Weybridge: (802) 545-2230

For Vermont-raised meats, including lamb, venison, rabbit, and quail, as well as other Vermont-grown or -raised ingredients:

- Vermont Fresh Network's searchable database at www.vermontfresh.net

For Vermont apples:

- Vermont Apple Marketing Board: www.vermontapples.org
- Shelburne Orchards, Shelburne: (802) 985-2753 or www.shelburne orchards.com

For Vermont breweries, cideries, and wineries:

- Vermont Brewers Association: www.vermontbrewers.com

Other sources for specific ingredients:

- For smoked sweet Spanish paprika and dried chiles de arbol, The Spice House: (312) 274-0378 or www.thespicehouse.com
- For wild ginger *(Asarum canadense),* try herbal stores in your area or Purple Shutter Herbs: (888) 865-4372
- For Merguez lamb sausage and non-Vermont game, including rabbit, duck, and venison, D'Artagnan: (800) 327-8246 or www.dartagnan.com
- For a variety of fresh and dried wild mushrooms, Aux Délices de Bois: (888) 547-5471 or www.auxdelices.com

Books

This is a brief list of books that Rick and Melissa found educational and inspirational while writing this cookbook:

Aidells, Bruce, and Denis Kelly. *The Complete Meat Book*. Boston: Houghton Mifflin, 1998.

Bentley, Virginia Williams. *The Bentley Farm Cookbook*. Boston: Houghton Mifflin, 1975.

Colicchio, Tom. *Craft of Cooking*. New York: Clarkson Potter, 2003.

English, Todd, and Sally Sampson. *The Olives Table*. New York: Simon & Schuster, 1997.

Fearnley-Whittingstall, Hugh. *The River Cottage Meat Book*. London: Hodder and Stoughton, 2004.

Kent, Louise Andrews. *The Vermont Year-Round Cookbook*. Boston: Houghton Mifflin, 1966.

Kunz, Gray. *The Elements of Taste*. New York: Little, Brown and Company, 2001.

Lawrence, James and Rux Martin. *Sweet Maple*. Montpelier and Shelburne: Vermont Life and Chapters, 1993.

Lincoff, Gary H. *National Audubon Society Field Guide to Mushrooms: North America*. New York: Knopf, 1981.

Raichlen, Steven. *How to Grill*. New York: Workman, 2001.

And for historical context and information on Shelburne Farms:

Dodge, Bertha S. *Tales of Vermont Ways and People*. Harrisburg, PA: Stackpole Books, 1977.

Donnis, Erica. Manuscript in progress on the history of Shelburne Farms.

Klyza, Christopher McGrory, and Stephen C. Trombulak. *The Story of Vermont: A Natural and Cultural History*. Hanover, NH: University Press of New England, 1999.

Lipke, William. *Shelburne Farms: The History of an Agricultural Estate.* Burlington, VT: University of Vermont, 1979.

Parella, Deborah. S*helburne Farms Project Seasons: Hands-on Activities for Discovering the Wonders of the World.* Shelburne, VT: Shelburne Farms, 1995.

Sherman, Joe. *The House at Shelburne Farms.* Forest Dale, VT: Paul S. Erickson, 1986.

Resources

About Shelburne Farms

Located along the shores of Lake Champlain in northwestern Vermont, Shelburne Farms started in 1886 as the model agricultural estate of William Seward Webb and Lila Osgood Vanderbilt Webb. From the beginning, it was a grand experiment designed to demonstrate new techniques in land use and farming. In 1972, family descendants established an independent 501(c)(3) education organization with the dream of using the Farm's resources to make a significant contribution to global environmental conservation. In 1984, the property was donated to the nonprofit, and it was designated as a National Historic Landmark in 2001.

Today Shelburne Farms is a working farm and vibrant education center dedicated to cultivating a conservation ethic by teaching and demonstrating the stewardship of natural and agricultural resources. As a living classroom visited by thousands of children, educators, and families each year, the 1,400-acre campus integrates education, agriculture, forestry, historic preservation, and community and cultural activities. Through innovative land use and restoration practices, hands-on education programs, its award-winning publication *Project Seasons,* and national and international partnerships, Shelburne Farms has become a source of inspiration for environmental stewardship and sustainable development locally and around the world.

Those who come to Shelburne Farms to enjoy the walking trails, attend an event, take a tour, stay at the historic Inn, or enjoy local food in its restaurant will gain insight into the rewards of stewardship and sustainable land use in a setting of exceptional natural and architectural beauty.

Shelburne Farms welcomes more than 120,000 visitors every year. The nonprofit organization is supported by gifts and grants from contributors all across the country, program and event fees, farm product sales (led by the award-winning Shelburne Farms cheddar cheese), and revenue from the restaurant and overnight accommodations at The Inn at Shelburne Farms.

To become a member of Shelburne Farms or for more information on its programs, products, and services, please contact:

Shelburne Farms
1611 Harbor Road, Shelburne, Vermont 05482
(802) 985-8686
www.shelburnefarms.org

Vermont and National Food and Farming Education Resources

Agriculture in the Classroom	www.agclassroom.org *Helps students gain a greater awareness of the role of agriculture in the economy and society (a USDA program)*
American Cheese Society	www.cheesesociety.org *Serves as an educational resource for cheesemakers and the public*
Center for Ecoliteracy	www.ecoliteracy.org *Promotes education for sustainable living*
Eat Well Guide	www.eatwellguide.org *Lists farms, stores, farmers' markets, and restaurants across the country that sell sustainably raised meat, eggs, and dairy products*
Edible Communities	www.ediblecommunities.com *Connects consumers with local growers, retailers, chefs, and food artisans*
Farm-Based Education Association	www.farmbasededucation.org *Nurtures and promotes farm-based education*

Farmers' markets nationwide	www.ams.usda.gov/farmersmarkets/map.htm *Lists farmers' markets in each state*
Food Education Every Day (FEED)	www.vtfeed.org *Takes a community-based approach to school food system change in Vermont*
Food Routes Network	www.foodroutes.org *Works to rebuild local, community-based food systems*
Grass-Fed Food Sources	www.eatwild.com *Lists pasture-based farms throughout the country that sell meat, eggs, butter, and cheese to the consumer*
Humane Farm Animal Care	www.certifiedhumane.org *Administers the Certified Humane Program, which inspects producers and processors*
Local Harvest	www.localharvest.org *Lists markets and restaurants throughout the country that specialize in locally grown food*
National Farm to School Program	www.farmtoschool.org *Connects schools with local farms to encourage the serving of healthy meals in school cafeterias, provision of health and nutrition education, and support of local farmers*
Northeast Organic Farming Association of Vermont	www.nofavt.org *Lists organic farms, farmers' markets, and community-supported agriculture farms, and includes many other useful links*
Renewing America's Food Traditions (RAFT)	www.environment.nau.edu/raft/ *Works to rescue America's diverse foods and food traditions (coalition of food, agriculture, conservation, and education organizations)*
Slow Food USA	www.slowfoodusa.org *Supports and celebrates the food traditions of North America*
Vermont Agency of Agriculture	www.vermontagriculture.com/agorgs.htm *Lists producers' associations and farmers' markets in Vermont*
Vermont Agriculture in the Classroom	www.vermontagriculture.com/AITC/ *Creates educational networks that promote farms, food production, nutrition, and resource management in Vermont communities*

Vermont Cheese Council	www.vtcheese.com	*Educates the public on the high quality and diversity of Vermont cheeses*
Vermont Eat Local Movement	www.eatlocalvt.org	*Works to broaden awareness and facilitate use of local foods in Chittenden County. (See the "cool links" page for other regional Eat Local groups.)*
Vermont Fresh Network	www.vermontfresh.net	*Builds partnerships among farmers, chefs, and consumers*
Vermont Institute for Artisan Cheese, University of Vermont	www.uvm.edu/viac	*Provides education, research, technical services, and public outreach to increase knowledge and appreciation of artisan cheese*

Acknowledgments

Melissa
would like to thank:

Amy for planting the idea.

Everyone at Shelburne Farms, especially Hilary.

Kitty and the Viking Studio team for falling in love with Shelburne Farms and bringing our book to life.

Susie and Jordan and their crews for capturing the food, the Farm, and the people so perfectly on film.

My intrepid recipe testers: Beth, Emily, and Millissa, plus Alexis, Christine, Deborah, Katie, and Liz.

All the Vermont farmers, cheesemakers, fruit growers, foragers, hunters, sugarmakers, bakers, butchers, cooks, and chefs who have educated and inspired me over the last six years—with special thanks to those who are in the book.

Molly for all of your invaluable advice.

Ed and Becky for your support, even while I was too busy to write for you.

Polly for always being willing to help out.

Rick for sharing your recipes and being open to developing new ones, for teaching me so much, and for being patient while I chased you around the kitchen with measuring spoons.

Mark, Nikko, and Alex—my biggest supporters and (usually) willing taste testers.

Rick
would like to thank:

Sheila, Luke, and Miles, my favorite people to cook for.

All the farmers and food producers in Vermont for showing me what fresh and local really means.

Shelburne Farms, a constant source of inspiration and the most beautiful place in the world to work.

Todd, for being my culinary school after culinary school.

Melissa, for letting me be a part of this and teaching me a whole new way to cook.

Index

ale-braised kielbasa with sauerkraut, 175–76
almond(s):
  -maple brittle, 270
  in maple-nut granola, 258–59
  for sour cherry-chocolate cheesecakes, 250–51
apple(s), 209–31
  beet, and radish salad, 191
  -blackberry crisp, 223
  butter, and oven-roasted applesauce, 229–30
  cider vinaigrette, 218
  and cinnamon-sugar pancakes, 212
  -cranberry brown butter tart, 224–25
  pie and cinnamon pinwheels, 226–28
  -rhubarb chutney, 215
  roast chicken with sausages and, 173–74
  roasted, and plum parfaits, 221–22
  rosemary-scented cider granita, 231
  slivered brussels sprouts with bacon and, 196
  smoked turkey, and cheddar strata, baked, 213–14
  tart, duck breast with hard cider and, 140–41
  tea bread, honeyed, 219–20
  varieties, 211
applesauce and apple butter, oven-roasted, 229–30
artichokes, braised rabbit with capers, lemon, and, 136–37
arugula and cider-glazed squash salad, 194

bacon:
  Canadian, scalloped potatoes with mushrooms and, 118–19

cornmeal fried trout with sage and, 153–54
  rabbit, and turnip stew, 138–39
  slivered brussels sprouts with apple and, 196
  wilted dandelion greens with croutons and, 66–67
beet, apple, and radish salad, 191
beverages:
  Jamaican-style ginger ale, 75
  mint-lime soda, 75
  rhubarb-citrus soda: a Vermont spring tonic, 74
biscuits, cheddar and herb, 24
Bivins, Tom, 262
blackberry-apple crisp, 223
black pepper and maple chicken, 48–49
blondies, maple sugar, 264–65
blue cheese:
  -black pepper compound butter, 9
  celery root soup with, 190
  mushroom and kale lasagna with, 116–17
Brie, warm maple and tart cherry, 52
brittle, maple-almond, 270
brussels sprouts, slivered, with bacon and apple, 196
Buck, John, 134
butter(s):
  brown, apple-cranberry tart, 224–25
  compound, 8–10
  home-churned, 6–7
buttermilk:
  dressing, and other uses for, 25
  homemade, 12, 163
  -plum sherbet, 254
butternut squash puree or soup, maple-roasted, 202–3
butterscotch:

-maple pudding, 261
-maple sauce, 271

calf's liver with sage, shallots, and maple-vinegar sauce, 50–51
cantaloupe and ham chopped salad, 162–63
capers:
  braised rabbit with artichokes, lemon and, 136–37
  -parsley compound butter, 9
carrots:
  and rutabaga, quick pickled, 189
  and turnips, honey-glazed, 197–98
cauliflower, roasted, with golden raisins and pine nuts, 201
celery root soup with blue cheese, 190
cheddar cheese:
  baked apple, and smoked turkey strata, 213–14
  and deviled ham spread, 168
  and herb biscuits, 24–25
  for macaroni and cheese with ham and horseradish, 28–29
  smash, shepherd's pie with caramelized onions and, 99–101
  -tomato soup, 15–16
cheese, *see* milk and cheese, savory; *specific cheeses*
cheesecakes, sour cherry-chocolate, 250–51
cheese plate basics, 23
chicken:
  maple and black pepper, 48–49
  milk-braised, with sage and bay, 30–31
  roast, with sausages and apples, 173–74
  with roasted garlic and mushrooms, 122–23
chickpeas, spice-rubbed lamb chops with fennel, tomatoes and, 92

Index